Clinical Governance in General Dental Practice

Raj Rattan

Ruth Chambers

and

Gill Wakley

Foreword by

Kevin Lewis

Dental Director
Dental Protection Ltd

Radcliffe Medical Press

Radcliffe Medical Press Ltd
18 Marcham Road
Abingdon
Oxon OX14 1AA
United Kingdom

www.radcliffe-oxford.com
The Radcliffe Medical Press electronic catalogue and online ordering facility.
Direct sales to anywhere in the world.

British Library Cataloguing in Publication Data

A catalogue record for this book is available from the British Library.

ISBN 1 85775 935 4

Typeset by Advance Typesetting Ltd, Oxfordshire
Printed and bound by TJ International Ltd, Padstow, Cornwall

Contents

Foreword

Clinical governance is a concept that has been widely trailed throughout the healthcare field in recent years, and unfortunately this process has created an aura of mystery and complexity. Little wonder, then, that general dental practitioners and their teams have viewed the advent of clinical governance with great scepticism and suspicion, and its implementation as an intimidating prospect.

It is refreshing, then, to see clinical governance stripped down to its essential values – for it is a simple enough concept, if viewed as a set of guiding principles as opposed to a complex and endless list of extra jobs to find time for.

There is a lot for me to like about this book and I am delighted to commend it to my friends and colleagues in general dental practice. First, practitioners will warm to the fact that the guiding principles of clinical governance are those which have already served industry and the world of business exceptionally well, throughout the era of total quality management (TQM) and service excellence. Their value and effectiveness is proven, and they have stood the test of time and experience in businesses of all sizes. Practitioners like to know that things will work.

Second, it is written in a style which is inviting, and which takes down barriers and objections rather than creating them. Each section provides a persuasive invitation to discover more, and the case studies make it easy for practitioners and their staff to identify with the issues, which as a result become real rather than remote.

Third, I know from experience that busy practitioners are generally very appreciative when a lot of the legwork has already been done for them. In this respect, this book excels with its templates, easy-to-read checklists and action plans.

Paradoxically, one of the problems for clinical governance in its quest for enthusiastic acceptance by general dental practitioners, was its inclusion in the National Health Service Terms of Service. Practitioners tend to work on the assumption that anything that is included within Regulations cannot be entirely trusted.

Perhaps the greatest compliment one can pay to the authors is that they have made clinical governance so logical, attractive and achievable, that the perhaps natural resistance to any new 'Terms of Service' obligation, tends to evaporate very early in the text. Indeed, it seems such a good idea that it is strange that no-one had thought of it before. Of course, the thinly veiled secret is that a large number of people – indeed, very successful people – had not only thought of it before, but have been relying upon these very principles for years.

The key issues of accountability, of setting and auditing standards to secure quality improvement and to encourage the pursuit of excellence, are admirable enough, if perhaps a little too conceptual for the busy reader. But the nitty gritty of involving every member of staff, identifying areas for improvement and developing strategies to work on them, finding new ways to demonstrate the achievement of standards, and managing people, systems, processes, time and money in order to create a culture in which these targets can be achieved consistently, is practical, everyday stuff that dental practices can really sink their teeth into.

Any text designed for general dental practitioners that strays too far from the realms of reality and achievability is doomed to be consigned to the 'pending' tray to gather dust, or to the circular floor-mounted filing system in the corner of every dentist's office. The section on 'meaningful patient involvement' is one of the jewels in the crown of this text; for too long, successive Governments and the profession have been making plans for patients and the services they will receive, without actually asking the patient. Clinical governance is not a valuable concept in its own right – it becomes a valuable concept only if it helps to deliver what patients need and want.

This balanced and very readable text is as good a place to start as I can possibly imagine.

Kevin J Lewis BDS LDS RCS
September 2002

During 20 years in full-time general dental practice and a further 10 years practising part-time, Kevin Lewis developed a special interest in preventive dentistry and practice management. He has written two textbooks on dental practice management and has been the Associate Editor of *Dental Practice* in the UK since 1981. He has worked in the medico-legal field, with Dental Protection, since 1989, first on the Board of Directors, then as a dento-legal advisor, before being appointed Dental Director in 1998.

Preface

This book aims to bridge the gap between the theory and practice of clinical governance in general dental practice.

It draws on the priorities of the clinical governance agenda that is part of the big picture within the NHS, and is informed by the experience of running a multi-surgery general dental practice.

The pace of change in general dental practice continues unabated, and it is inevitable that the systems and processes which have been the backbone of successful general dental practice for many decades will need to evolve to mirror the new age.

Remuneration systems will need to be developed to reflect the new priorities of the NHS. It is inevitable that there will be a rethink about the training, education and integration of the dental workforce if they are to deliver a high quality of care in a way that meets the needs of patients.

Clinical governance will underpin the process of change by:

- sustaining quality improvements
- defining standards
- demonstrating achievements
- emphasising the need for continuous professional development.

The emphasis in this book is on doing rather than on theorising. There is some theory and there is also some jargon, since to remove this from the text would not only limit the scope of the work but also restrict its potential application.

General dental practitioners do not always approve of the propensity of the NHS towards jargon, but as there are wide-ranging changes on the horizon, the effective use of jargon is one way to facilitate the communication process between the providers and commissioners of services. We may as well start getting used to it.

In a remarkable book[1] on the challenges of sustaining momentum in learning organisations, the authors state that 'the business world today is gripped by tremendous cross-currents concerning the philosophy and practice of governance'. They note that in developing governance systems we should be 'prepared to receive, and feel, a great deal of emotional heat'. It is no different in dentistry.

I have some sympathy with this view, and I hope that this book helps to cool the emotions sufficiently to allow some objective interpretation of clinical governance in general dental practice.

Raj Rattan
September 2002

Reference

1   Senge P, Kleiner A, Roberts C *et al.* (1999) *The Dance of Change*. Nicholas Brealey Publishing, London.

About the authors

Raj Rattan is a dentist with over 20 years' experience of general dental practice. He now combines his practising career with running a dental vocational training scheme within the London Deanery, and he holds a number of advisory and consultancy positions for professional organisations, including Dental Protection Ltd, primary care trusts and the Department of Health. He is a member of the Faculty of General Dental Practitioners and a former examiner for the MFGDP examination. He has published a number of articles and books on various aspects of general dental practice, and has lectured extensively throughout the UK and overseas.

Raj has run and organised numerous workshops and presentations on aspects of clinical governance for local dental committees, health authorities, primary care trusts, Dental Bodies Corporate, Denplan and various postgraduate centres throughout the UK.

The views expressed in this book are those of the authors and do not necessarily reflect the views of the organisations to which Raj acts as an adviser or consultant.

Ruth Chambers has been a GP for 20 years. Her previous experience has encompassed a wide range of research and educational activities, including stress and the health of doctors, the quality of healthcare and many other topics.

She is currently the Professor of Primary Care Development at the School of Health at Staffordshire University. She was the Chair of Staffordshire Medical Audit Advisory Group and a GP trainer for many years. Ruth has initiated and run all types of educational initiatives and activities. She and Gill Wakley have run workshops to teach GPs, hospital consultants, nurses, therapists and non-clinical staff about clinical governance. The experiences of the workshops and how the participants put their learning about clinical governance into action inform this book.

Gill Wakley started in general practice in 1966, but transferred to community medicine shortly afterwards and then into public health. A desire for increased contact with patients caused a move back into general practice, together with community gynaecology, in 1978. She has been combining the two, in varying amounts, ever since.

Throughout, Gill has been heavily involved in learning and teaching. She was in a training general practice, became an instructing doctor and a regional assessor in family planning, and was until recently a senior clinical lecturer with the Primary Care Department at Keele University, Staffordshire. Like Ruth, she has run all types of educational initiatives and activities, from individual mentoring and instruction to small group work, plenary lectures, distance-learning programmes, workshops, and courses for a wide range of health professionals and lay people.

Acknowledgements

It has been my past experience that the writing of the 'Acknowledgements' page in any text occupies a disproportionate amount of time when compared with the rest of the work mainly because of the author's concerns about the risk of omission.

This book is the exception. It was the suggestion of my publishers to seek collaboration from Ruth Chambers, Professor of Primary Care Development at the School of Health at Staffordshire University, and Gill Wakley, General Medical Practitioner, whose book *Making Clinical Governance Work for You* had already been published by Radcliffe Medical Press to great acclaim.

Their co-operation and agreement to use the core text and format were immediately forthcoming, and I would like to put on record the fact that without their co-operation, encouragement and support this book would not have been written.

I would like to thank them for giving me the tools to reinvent this particular wheel.

Finally, I must also thank Bromley and Croydon Health Authorities (as they were then) for their support and encouragement of this project.

Raj Rattan
September 2002

List of abbreviations

BDA	British Dental Association	ISO	International Organisation for Standardisation
BDHF	British Dental Health Foundation	LDC	Local Dental Committee
CDS	Community Dental Service	NICE	National Institute for Clinical Excellence
CG	clinical governance	NSF	National Service Framework
CHC	Community Health Council	OHX	Oral Health Index
CHI	Commission for Health Improvement	PALS	patient advocacy and liaison service
CPD	continuing professional development	PCD	professionals complementary to dentistry
DPB	Dental Practice Board	PCT	primary care trust
DRO	Dental Reference Officer	PDS	Personal Dental Services
EDI	Electronic Data Interchange	PGEA	postgraduate education allowance
EHR	electronic health record	SWOT	strengths, weaknesses, opportunities and threats
FGDP	Faculty of General Dental Practitioners	TQM	total quality management
GDC	General Dental Council	WHO	World Health Organization
GDP	general dental practitioner		
GDS	General Dental Service		
HIMP	Health Improvement and Modernisation Plan		

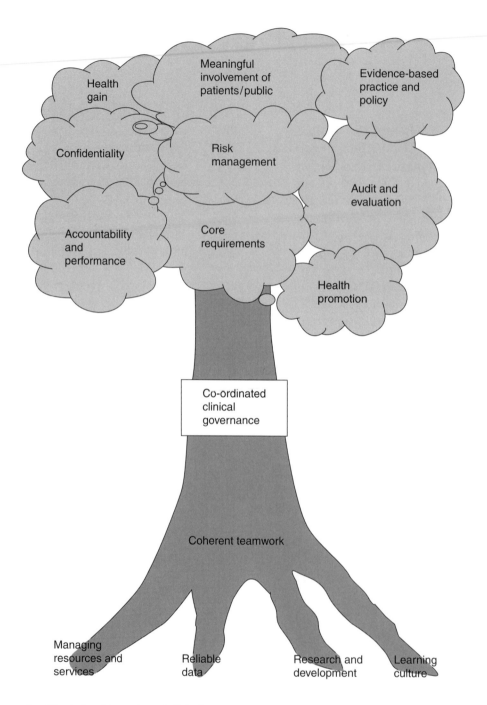

Figure A   'Routes' and branches of clinical governance.

PART ONE

Introduction

CHAPTER ONE

What's new?

On 18 March 1965, Russian cosmonaut Alexi Leonov became the first man to 'walk in space'. Attached by a ten-foot tether to Voskhod II, his 'space walk' lasted ten minutes and guaranteed him a permanent place in space history. The Americans responded three months later, and Ed White II did the honours on 3 June from Gemini IV. He, too, had 'walked in space'.

How things have changed. Astronauts no longer 'walk in space'. Instead they carry out extra-vehicular activities (EVAs). These EVAs are no longer limited to hovering by an umbilical and photographing the planet from space – they now carry toolkits so that they can fix things and show the world that they have come on a bit since those heady days of the 1960s.

Yet fundamentally the EVA is a space walk – it is a space walk with tools.

So it is with clinical governance. We have new words, which essentially reflect not so new concepts. The real problem in the perception of clinical governance among general dental practitioners (GDPs) is that the words have no 'intuitive meaning'.[1] Added to the woes of altered perception is the observation that the word 'governance' in the intended sense ('*the manner in which something is governed or regulated; method of management, system of regulations*') is marked as obsolete in the *Oxford English Dictionary*. The irony of this will not be lost on readers.

One definition of clinical governance describes it as 'a system through which NHS organisations are accountable for continuously improving the quality of their services and safeguarding high standards of care by creating an environment in which excellence in clinical care will flourish'.[2]

It is about finding ways 'to implement care that works in an environment in which clinical effectiveness can flourish by establishing a facilitatory culture'.[3]

The pillars of clinical governance

The clinical governance agenda is underpinned by core principles that are reflected in the 'tree model' of clinical governance shown on page xii and on which this text is based. The expression *pillars of clinical governance* is also often used to categorise the various focal points of the agenda and, depending on what you read, there are seven to ten pillars of clinical governance which reflect the underlying themes. The so-called ten pillars include the following elements:

1   evidence-based practice
2   dissemination of good ideas
3   quality improvement processes in place
4   high-quality data to monitor care
5   clinical risk reduction programmes
6   adverse events investigation
7   lessons learned from patient complaints
8   poor clinical performance tackled
9   professional development programmes
10 leadership skill development.

This summary is useful because it exposes the individual elements of the agenda. The disadvantage of working to a list like this is that it does not demonstrate the importance of integrating the different facets. An alternative presentation is proposed which not only clarifies the importance of integration of the individual elements, but also allows for their tailoring to suit practice circumstances and local PCT priorities.

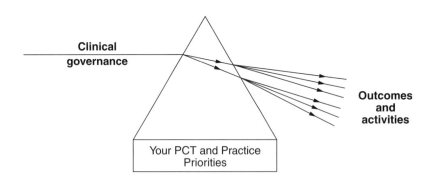

Figure 1.1   The Prism Effect: helping to implement the clinical governance agenda at local level.

The business of clinical governance

Clinical governance in primary dental care is nourished by the tenets of successful business practice. It draws on practice management principles, but applies additional tools to reflect and demonstrate to the rest of the world that we, like the astronauts, have moved on a bit as well. There are echoes of corporate governance, an initiative originally aimed at redressing failing standards in the business world through the Cadbury Report.[4]

Clinical governance and total quality management

The pillars of clinical governance are very similar to the building blocks of total quality management (TQM), which are as follows:

*   leadership
*   organisation
*   training
*   customer focus – internal and external
*   measurement
*   work processes
*   teamwork
*   communication
*   planning
*   recognition.

TQM has been defined as 'a process designed to focus on customer expectations, the prevention of problems, building commitment to continuous improvement in everyone and the promotion of participative management'.[5]

Clinical governance aims to unite managerial, organisational and clinical approaches to improving quality of care. This relationship is established in the quality improvement processes that drive clinical governance in a remarkably similar way to the processes that drive business.

Clinical governance and the ISO

The International Organisation for Standardisation (ISO) has been developing voluntary technical standards over almost all sectors of business, industry and technology since 1947. ISO 9000 was introduced in 1987. The new standard, ISO 9001:2000, was introduced in December 2000, and it differed from the 1994 standard in its emphasis on increased management involvement in the quality process (the absence of this was a major criticism of the 1994 standard).

The quality management principles for the revised ISO 9001:2000 are intended to be 'used by senior management as a framework to guide their organisations towards improved performance'.[6] The definition bears a remarkable similarity to that of clinical governance in the 1998 White Paper.

The quality principles and the potential benefits are summarised here and reproduced by kind permission of ISO, Geneva.

Principle 1: Customer focus

Organisations depend on their customers and should therefore understand current and future customer needs, meet customer requirements and strive to exceed customer expectations.

The key benefits are as follows:

- increased revenue and market share obtained through flexible and fast responses to market opportunities
- increased effectiveness in the use of the organisation's resources to enhance customer satisfaction
- improved customer loyalty leading to repeat business.

Applying the principle of customer focus typically leads to:

- researching and understanding customer needs and expectations
- ensuring that the objectives of the organisation are linked to customer needs and expectations
- communicating customer needs and expectations throughout the organisation
- measuring customer satisfaction and acting on the results
- systematically managing customer relationships
- ensuring a balanced approach with regard to satisfying customers and other interested parties (e.g. owners, employees, suppliers, financiers, local communities and society as a whole).

Principle 2: Leadership

Leaders establish unity of purpose and direction of the organisation. They should create and maintain the internal environment in which people can become fully involved in achieving the organisation's objectives.

The key benefits are as follows:

- people will understand and be motivated towards the organisation's goals and objectives
- activities are evaluated, aligned and implemented in a unified way
- miscommunication between the different levels of the organisation will be minimised.

Applying the principle of leadership typically leads to:

- considering the needs of all interested parties, including customers, owners, employees, suppliers, financiers, local communities and society as a whole
- establishing a clear vision of the organisation's future
- setting challenging goals and targets
- creating and sustaining shared values, fairness and ethical role models at all levels of the organisation
- establishing trust and eliminating fear

- providing people with the resources, training and freedom necessary for them to act with responsibility and accountability
- inspiring, encouraging and recognising people's contributions.

Principle 3: Involvement of people

People at all levels represent the essence of an organisation, and their full involvement enables their abilities to be used for the organisation's benefit.

The key benefits are as follows:

- motivated, committed and involved people within the organisation
- innovation and creativity in furthering the organisation's objectives
- people being accountable for their own performance
- people eager to participate in and contribute to continual improvement.

Applying the principle of involvement of people typically leads to:

- people understanding the importance of their contribution to, and role in, the organisation
- people identifying constraints on their performance
- people accepting ownership of problems and their responsibility for solving them
- people evaluating their performance against their personal goals and objectives
- people actively seeking opportunities to enhance their competence, knowledge and experience
- people freely sharing their knowledge and experience
- people openly discussing problems and issues.

Principle 4: Process approach

A desired result is achieved more efficiently when activities and related resources are managed as a process.

The key benefits are as follows:

- lower costs and shorter cycle times through effective use of resources
- improved, consistent and predictable results
- focused and prioritised improvement opportunities.

Applying the principle of process approach typically leads to:

- systematically defining the activities necessary to obtain a desired result
- establishing clear responsibility and accountability for managing key activities
- analysing and measuring the capability of key activities
- identifying the interfaces of key activities within and between the functions of the organisation
- focusing on the factors (e.g. resources, methods, materials) that will improve key activities of the organisation

- evaluating risks, consequences and the impact of activities on customers, suppliers and other interested parties.

Principle 5: *System approach to management*

Identifying, understanding and managing interrelated processes as a system contributes to the organisation's effectiveness and efficiency in achieving its objectives.

The key benefits are as follows:

- integration and alignment of the processes that will best achieve the desired results
- ability to focus effort on the key processes
- giving interested parties confidence in the consistency, effectiveness and efficiency of the organisation.

Applying the principle of system approach to management typically leads to:

- structuring a system to achieve the organisation's objectives in the most effective and efficient way
- understanding the interdependencies between the different processes of the system
- structured approaches that harmonise and integrate processes
- providing a better understanding of the roles and responsibilities necessary to achieve common objectives and thereby reduce cross-functional barriers
- understanding organisational capabilities and establishing resource constraints prior to action
- targeting and defining how specific activities within a system should operate
- continually improving the system through measurement and evaluation.

Principle 6: *Continual improvement*

Continual improvement of the organisation's overall performance should be a permanent objective of the organisation.

The key benefits are as follows:

- performance advantage through improved organisational capabilities
- alignment of improvement activities at all levels with the organisation's strategic intent
- flexibility necessary to react quickly to opportunities.

Applying the principle of continual improvement typically leads to:

- employing a consistent organisation-wide approach to continual improvement of the organisation's performance
- providing people with training in the methods and tools of continual improvement
- making continual improvement of products, processes and systems an objective for every individual in the organisation

- establishing goals to guide and measures to track continual improvement
- recognising and acknowledging improvements.

Principle 7: *Factual approach to decision making*

Effective decisions are based on the analysis of data and information.
The key benefits are as follows:

- informed decisions
- an increased ability to demonstrate the effectiveness of past decisions by reference to factual records
- increased ability to review, challenge and change opinions and decisions.

Applying the principle of factual approach to decision making typically leads to:

- ensuring that data and information are sufficiently accurate and reliable
- making data accessible to those who need them
- analysing data and information using valid methods
- making decisions and taking action based on factual analysis, balanced by experience and intuition.

Principle 8: *Mutually beneficial supplier relationships*

An organisation and its suppliers are interdependent, and a mutually beneficial relationship enhances the ability of both to create value.
The key benefits are as follows:

- increased ability to create value for both parties
- flexibility and speed of joint responses to changing market or customer needs and expectations
- optimisation of costs and resources.

Applying the principles of mutually beneficial supplier relationships typically leads to:

- establishing relationships that balance short-term gains against long-term considerations
- pooling of expertise and resources with partners
- identifying and selecting key suppliers
- clear and open communication
- sharing information and future plans
- establishing joint development and improvement activities
- inspiring, encouraging and recognising improvements and achievements by suppliers.

In a review of the acceptance of this standard, it was described as a 'significant step in the right direction towards a more holistic business approach to quality'.[7]
It is the same for clinical governance.

Clinical governance and the World Health Organization

The World Health Organization (WHO) divides clinical governance into four aspects:[8]

1 professional performance
2 resource use (efficiency)
3 risk management
4 patients' satisfaction with the service provided.

As you can see, the same themes are reflected within the core aspects.

Clinical governance and the Commission for Health Improvement

To reinforce further the shared principles, you may want to consider each of the bullet points in the Commission for Health Improvement (CHI) model and adapt them to your current views about good practice management. Here are some examples from some of the leaders in management thinking.

The CHI model (*see* Figure 1.2) reflects the belief of the CHI that effective clinical governance depends on the following:

1 a culture of continuous learning
2 innovations which improve patient care
3 improving patients' experiences
4 improving outcomes
5 strategic development of the service so that it focuses on patients.

It is interesting to compare these with the widely recognised benefits of TQM, which are as follows:

1 an increase in productivity
2 improved services to customers
3 improved bottom-line profit
4 greater business efficiency
5 business priorities focused on the needs of the customer.

The emphasis may vary, but the similarities are self-evident.

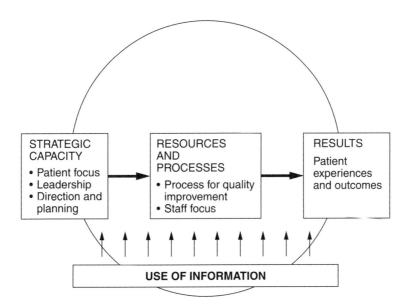

Figure 1.2   The CHI model of clinical governance.

Conflict

Is there a conflict between the provision of high-quality services for patients and the financial needs of the business? Practices need to be profitable in order to improve the quality of care for patients. Sometimes this can cause frustration in general dental practice, but balancing the demands of clinical practice and business practice has always been a challenge for dentists in general dental practice. We may not relish the thought, but we have to grapple with these issues every day in general practice.

In response to a letter in the *British Dental Journal*, the editor wrote 'I regret to say that the influences of the competitive market do apply to the dental profession. We may not like this fact, but it remains true.'[9]

The challenge for dentists is to take the clinical governance agenda, review its purpose and align it with practice development. We know that improving outcomes and enhancing patients' experiences make for value-added dentistry. And as small businesses, we know that this helps to promote loyalty to the practice, and it encourages practice growth and profit. This business model is reflected on the front cover of one of the leading texts on business management, *The Service Profit Chain*, which sets out to describe how companies 'link profit and growth to loyalty, satisfaction and value'.

This relationship is shown in Figure 1.3.

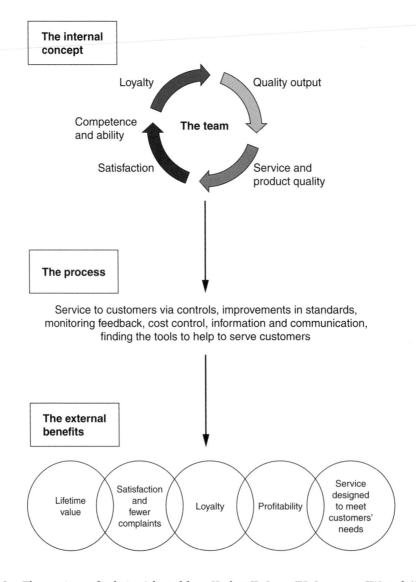

Figure 1.3   The service profit chain. Adapted from Heskett JL, Jones TO, Loveman GW *et al.* (1994) Putting the service profit chain to work. *Harvard Business Rev.* 166.

Making it happen

Clinical governance is a developmental process and it will evolve over a decade. We hope we have demonstrated that its roots are embedded in concepts which are already familiar to GDPs. To carry the agenda forward, it has been suggested that it 'builds on (these) elements with which practitioners are familiar'.[10]

This view is reflected in the British Dental Association's factsheet on the subject, which states that 'every practice already has the essentials of a clinical governance system, with someone in charge and established work processes. The question is – are responsibilities and accountability clear enough, and are processes consistently enough observed?'[11]

So, put simply, clinical governance 'is doing anything and everything required to maximise quality'.[12] It is about finding ways to 'implement care that works in an environment in which clinical effectiveness can flourish by establishing a facilitatory culture'.[3] The idea is to be more systematic about the way in which we do things, and to try to mesh with the big picture that is healthcare in its broadest sense.

In its journal to members, one of the medical advisers to the Medical and Dental Defence Union of Scotland wrote that it was important 'to emphasise that much of what is expected of doctors and dentists is already part of their daily practice'. He concluded that the real challenge was to make 'more explicit those aspirations to high standards and continuous quality improvement that they had already set for themselves'.[13]

A team effort

The quality of the workforce dictates the quality of the healthcare that they deliver. An effective workforce is one in which individuals are competent to carry out their current roles and responsibilities, and in which their training anticipates new models of service delivery. Achieving this requires adequate resources and the right learning environment throughout the health service.

Clinical governance underpins this way of working and accounting for the following:

- sustaining quality improvements
- minimising inequalities in access to dental services for different groups of the population
- reducing variations in healthcare services
- defining standards
- demonstrating achievements.

The emphasis in this book is on what individuals and workplace teams themselves can do first to identify their own learning needs, and then to draw up and prioritise their own action plans.

The material is based around 14 themes as core components of a quality healthcare service. The idea is to try to overcome the gulf that exists between theory and practice, or between talking about something and actually doing it.

The emphasis is on education and training programmes being relevant to service needs, whether at practice or individual levels. 'Continuing professional development (CPD) programmes need to meet both the learning needs of individual health professionals to inspire public confidence in their skills ... and the wider service development needs of the NHS.'[2] CPD is not just what you *want* to do, but what you *need* to do.

Lifelong learning and continuing professional development are an integral part of clinical governance. Everyone should have learning goals that are relevant to service development.

In this book, we have identified 14 themes as core components of professional and service development which, taken together, constitute *clinical governance* – *see* Figure A, p. xii. These are as follows:

1   learning culture – in your practice
2   research and development culture
3   reliable data
4   well-managed resources and services, as individuals, as a team and as a practice
5   coherent team – well-integrated teamwork in the practice
6   meaningful involvement of patients and the public
7   health gain – activities to improve the health of patients
8   confidentiality – of information in consultations, in medical notes, and between practitioners
9   evidence-based practice and policy – applying it in practice
10 accountability and performance – for standards, performance of individuals, performance of practice
11 core requirements – good fit between skill mix and competence, communication, workforce numbers, morale in practice
12 health promotion – for patients
13 audit and evaluation – when making changes and assessing performance
14 risk management – proactive review, follow-up, risk management and risk reduction.

The big picture

In recent times there has been an increasing awareness of and desire to bring dentistry into the big picture that is the NHS – *see* Figure 1.4. It is part of the Government's programme of modernisation of the health services which sets out to:[2]

•   tackle the causes of ill health
•   make services convenient, quick and easy to use
•   ensure the consistency of services regardless of where a person lives
•   try to provide 'joined-up' services that are not constrained by artificial barriers between services, such as health and social services
•   invest in improving the workforce and infrastructure.[12]

It is hoped to achieve this through the following:[14]

•   clear national standards set by the National Service Frameworks (NSFs) and the National Institute for Clinical Excellence (NICE)

- local delivery of quality services
- monitoring of services through the Commission for Health Improvement (CHI)
- consultation with patients and the public.

Clinical governance is relevant to all five aims, and integral to the delivery of high-quality services in consultation with patients and the public at large. Minimising inequalities is at the heart of clinical governance:

- as inequalities in healthcare – variations in access, service provision or standards of care, and discrimination on the grounds of age, gender, ethnicity, sexuality, disability, etc.
- as inequalities of people's health – influenced by risky lifestyles and by social determinants of health, such as poor housing, low income, lack of transport.

We have established that the components of clinical governance are not new. However, bringing them together under the banner of clinical governance is a way of introducing more explicit accountability for performance.

Developments in primary dental care must take heed of the big picture, and will need to be consistent with the wider priorities. You may wonder why some issues have been discussed in this text which at first sight may not appear to be relevant to everyday practice (e.g. issues relating to patient-held records). The reason is that they are part of the big picture, and it is important that we as GDPs have an understanding not only of what is current but also of what may be around the corner. This is why we shall sometimes refer back to the big picture scenario.

Carefully evaluating your work and subsequent improvements in patient care will enable you to form your own view about the place of clinical governance in your practice.

The footprints of clinical governance

When the Americans put men on the moon, the world stood still, and a few years ago the world joined NASA and the crew of Apollo 11 to celebrate the thirtieth anniversary of that historic first landing.

However, the sceptics were less inclined to join in. Their concerns remained unanswered. Where, they continued to ask, was the real evidence to support the view that man had actually landed on the moon? Their belief is still that the entire episode had been secretly filmed in the Nevada Desert.

We suggest that the evidence is there. Someone just needs to go and have a look, because Messrs Armstrong and Aldrin would have left some footprints behind.

It is the same with clinical governance. We know that many of the processes are already happening in general dental practice. What we now need to do is to provide the footprints of evidence.

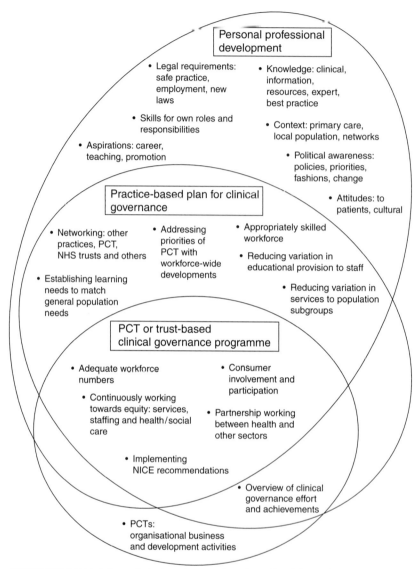

Note: The topics given as priority areas for development are examples, and are not intended to constitute comprehensive lists.

Figure 1.4   The components of professional development and how they fit in with the big picture.

References

1   Goodman NW (1998) Clinical governance. *BMJ*. **317**: 1725–7.

2   Department of Health (1998) *A First-Class Service: quality in the new NHS*. Department of Health, London.

3   Chambers R and Wall D (2000) *Teaching Made Easy: a manual for health professionals.* Radcliffe Medical Press, Oxford.

4   Committee on Financial Aspects of Corporate Governance (1992) *Report.* Gee, London.

5   Prism Consultants; www.prismcon.com

6   www.iso.ch

7   Daniel FJ (2001) *ISO 9001:2000 – Direct Hit?* Institute of Quality Assurance, London.

8   World Health Organization (1983) *The Principles of Quality Assurance.* World Health Organization, Copenhagen.

9   Grace M (1997) Editor's response to letter. *Br Dent J.* **183**: 239.

10 Audrey C (1999) Clinical governance in the GDS. *DPB Magazine.* **Nov**: 20–1, 36.

11 British Dental Association (2001) *Clinical Governance in General Dental Practice.* BDA factfile. March 2001. BDA, London.

12 Lilley R (1999) *Making Sense of Clinical Governance.* Radcliffe Medical Press, Oxford.

13 Rodger J (1999) *J Med Dent Defence Union Scot.* **Spring**: 1.

14 Department of Health (1997) *The New NHS: modern, dependable.* The Stationery Office, London.

CHAPTER TWO

How to do it: identify your practice development needs and your associated learning needs

Get organised as an individual

1   A useful starting point is to look at what plans you have for practice development in the short and medium term. From these you can create a practice development plan. Your own professional development could be part of this big picture. Regard your own plan as contributing to the wider practice-based clinical governance programme. You will need to consider the time commitment, the wider professional perspectives, motivation, prioritisation and support from the team, as well as the current requirements of the General Dental Council (GDC) and those in the General Dental Service (GDS) Regulations.

2   Identify the learning and training needs of the members of your team. Find the balance between the needs of individuals and those of your practice (e.g. patient service training or additional training to understand the systems that operate in your practice).

3   Devise a programme that meets these needs and fits with the priorities for *your* practice.

4   Select the resource material necessary to facilitate this process.

5   Appraise your own learning and professional development, and what you have achieved in improvements to patient care. Get feedback from others.

6   Review the practice/professional interface – demonstrate that your working environment is fit for you to practise from. Practice visit checklists are a useful starting point.

7   Identify new areas of learning and development from your self-evaluation exercise. Anticipate your own needs if your practising circumstances are about to change for any reason.

Some ideas

You could use the simple but effective *threes* format and involve your practice team in the same way. You could include the following idea in a simple questionnaire for each of them.

- Think of *three* areas in which you are confident and can do well.
- Think of *three* areas that you would like to know about.
- Think of *three* areas that you know nothing about.
- From these, choose *three* areas which one needs to know about in order to be good at what you do.
- Identify a specific objective in each of those *three* areas to improve your practice.

Get organised as a practice

1   Start with the business plan of your practice. If there is no business plan, consider drawing one up. What are the main areas you want to develop for the forthcoming year? Look further ahead at your medium-term plans. What about the next three years?

2   Identify service development needs and staff learning needs using some of the range of methods that follow in the next section. What are the main areas of planned development for which you and other staff will need new knowledge and skills? Consider checking with others from outside the practice whether you have got it right. Try to define short-term objectives for learning and development as well as taking a medium-term approach for, say, three to five years.

3   Identify what your team members need to learn to be able to deliver your clinical governance development programme. Balance clinical and non-clinical needs between individuals and their working environment. This will include:

   - generic learning that is relevant for everyone (e.g. communication)
   - teambuilding
   - specific skills for the particular roles and responsibilities of team members.

4   Assess the infrastructure required to deliver your planned clinical governance programme, and identify from where you will obtain the necessary resources.

5   When making your overall clinical governance plan you will need to consider the following:

   - which staff it covers – ideally it should include everyone
   - the extent of their commitment
   - their perspectives
   - how to motivate the team
   - how to prioritise development between topics, between different services or practices and between staff

- how to support the staff through changes
- how to evaluate what has been achieved
- how to assess and meet learning and service development needs as they occur.

Try to give each member of staff a definite role and responsibility in the overall plan. Think how and by whom the learning and clinical governance effort will be evaluated and achievements monitored, and how and by whom new learning needs will be identified and included.

6   Make it happen in practice.
7   Demonstrate that your working environment is fit for the staff to practise in, with good records of what you have achieved (e.g. improvements in the quality of patient care, staff morale, effective systems, staff development).
8   Evaluate the extent and quality of the service developments and associated learning, and describe what has still to be addressed.

You may find the grid in Table 2.1 helpful in achieving this.

Table 2.1 Your clinical governance plan

		Notes
Business plan	What is your plan?	What areas are a priority?
Service development	What areas of the service do you want to develop? List them as clinical and non-clinical areas	
Staff development	Who are the members of your team? List them and their job titles	What knowledge and skills do they need to develop?
Resources	What are you going to need by way of support?	Where could you seek this support?
What is your clinical governance plan?	Where do you want to start? How will you get the team on board?	Who could you approach for additional help?
Look at the practice environment	List the areas that you think could be improved upon	What is the evidence to support its suitability as a practising environment?
Extent and quality of service	What are the issues that still need to be addressed?	Look at the route/branch model of clinical governance and make a list of your concerns

What methods could you use to identify your practice development and learning needs?

There are many ways in which you can do this. You may want to review the options shown below and use one or more combinations that best suit your practice and your personal preferences.

1 Self-appraisal and peer appraisal

Your and your practice's aspirations for:

- new models of service delivery
- new roles and responsibilities within the practice
- your vision for the practice.

Your attitudes to:

- other disciplines
- patients
- lifelong learning
- culture
- change.

Your knowledge of:

- clinical techniques
- local demographics and trends
- current good practice guidelines
- the range of other dental services available locally
- systems and procedures

- business and management skills
- inequalities in service provision
- the wider issues within the NHS which may impact on your practice's future development.

Legal requirements:

- legislation on health and safety at work
- new legislation
- employment law.

Awareness of health policies:

- new health policies
- national priorities
- local priorities
- trends in clinical practice.

Skills:

- teamworking and communication
- development of the team
- effective working practices
- your competence in carrying out different clinical procedures.

2 Ask other people what they think of you: gain feedback from colleagues

Workshops, individual mentoring, small groups or just talking with colleagues about how you do your job all help you to assess your needs.

The first (and then experimental) peer review schemes funded by the Department of Health proved to be very popular. Those dentists who took part found the process valuable from both a personal and a professional perspective. The fact that many of those early groups continue to meet on a regular basis and continue to attract more participants to discuss issues of topical interest is testament to the value of the process.

Unless there is a method of recording the learning needs for yourself and your team, you will easily forget them in the busy environment of the dental practice.

One approach is to identify problems as they arise and to treat them as learning opportunities. This approach has the advantage of addressing real-life challenges in real-life situations which makes the outcomes more acceptable and relevant. This approach is particularly useful in induction training for new members of the dental team, but it is also worth considering for longstanding team members.

3 Select an audit (*see* Module 9 on Audit and evaluation)

Set standards for your performance and compare them with best practice, make changes and re-audit. Choose a topic where changes will make a significant difference to patient care.

- *Patient record card analysis.* This provides an insight into current recorded practice. Select a number of cards at random and look for possible inconsistencies in the way in which information is recorded, and review clinical procedures in light of your findings.
- *Peer review.* Compare an area of work with that of another individual, or compare work teams.
- *Criteria-based audit.* This compares clinical practice with specific standards, guidelines or protocols. Re-audit of changes should demonstrate improvements in the quality of care.
- *External audit.* The Dental Practice Board (DPB) has statistical data on your NHS clinical treatment patterns. Review the DPB profile with those of others in the practice.
- *Direct observation.* Record what is observed for later action – make a note of events as they occur – before you forget!
- *Surveys.* You might conduct a survey among your patients as a general indicator of care or for detecting a problem, but remember that it is a rather subjective measure of performance.
- *Significant event audit.* Think of a critical incident in which a patient or you experienced an adverse event.

Significant event audit is a very useful tool, and it can be applied to a clinical or non-clinical situation. The sequence of activities is summarised by the following six-step model.

- *Step 1.* Describe the critical incident – who, what, when.
- *Step 2.* Recount the effects of the event on the participants and the professionals involved.
- *Step 3.* Deduce the reasons for the critical event or situation arising, through discussion with other colleagues, review of case notes or other records.
- *Step 4.* Decide how you or others might have behaved differently, and describe your options with regard to how the procedures at work might be changed to reduce or eliminate reoccurrence.
- *Step 5.* Agree any changes that are needed, how they will be implemented, who will be responsible for what and when.
- *Step 6.* Re-audit at a later date to see whether changes to procedures are having the desired effects. Give feedback to the practice team. Acknowledge good care.

4 Monitor your own or your practice's clinical care

- Use DPB prescribing profiles or computer-generated data on treatment provision as a discussion item at practice meetings.
- Collate dental reference office reports and compare and contrast the outcomes of Dental Reference Officer examinations.
- Review the extent to which you adhere to clinical protocols, guidelines and evidence-based care.
- Identify any shortfalls in the provision of care and services.

5 Monitor access, availability and satisfaction

Access and availability

- Look at your opening hours.
- Could accessibility to the premises be improved?
- You could look at how close to their appointed time patients are seen by using either computerised appointment lists or pen and paper to record the time of arrival, the time of the appointment, and the actual time at which the patient was seen.
- You could look at next available appointments.
- You could review your appointment system to see if there are ways of prioritising care (e.g. emergency slots in the appointment book).
- Then you could compare the results after a selected time interval and see how what changes have taken place.

Patient satisfaction and referrals

- *Patient satisfaction.* Patient satisfaction surveys are one way of finding out what patients think of you. They have their shortcomings, but they will provide you with another footprint of clinical governance. Other ways to involve patients include the use of suggestion boxes, and keeping accurate records of all complaints, however trivial they may appear at first glance. Consider looking for patterns and/or trends in the comments received.
- *Referrals to the Community Dental Service/hospitals/specialists and other agencies.* You can audit whether referrals are appropriate by the use of pro formas or templates.

6 Monitoring systems and procedures

Regular problems need action and reviews. Regular team meetings can flag up such problems at an early stage. Do not be overly concerned if all of the difficulties cannot be resolved immediately. You may need to seek more information before planning action.

Monitoring systems need to be in place for all equipment and surgery supplies. Again this is an essential facet of good and effective practice management. It is worth having a separate file for recording the purchase of major equipment, and noting the arrangements for servicing and responsibility for maintenance. Remember to include a back-up option or deputy arrangements in case of absence or sickness.

Staff health records need to be checked as well, and robust systems must be put in place (e.g. to check hepatitis B status periodically). Be especially careful when employing locum or temporary staff, or with initial employment.

7 Informal conversations

It is often said that people learn most on courses when chatting with colleagues at the coffee and meal breaks. This is when you realise that other people are doing things differently to you – and if they seem to be doing them better and achieving more, you can challenge yourself to decide whether this matter could be one of your blind spots.

8 Strengths, weaknesses, opportunities and threats (SWOT) analysis

This is a tried and tested management tool. Undertake a SWOT analysis of your own performance or that of your practice team. You could do this on your own or with a work colleague or a peer group.

Strengths and weaknesses of individual practitioners might include any of the following:

- knowledge
- experience
- expertise
- research skills
- interprofessional relationships
- communication skills
- political skills
- organisational skills
- decision making
- timekeeping
- teaching skills.

Strengths and weaknesses of the practice organisation might relate to most of these aspects, too, as well as to resources (staff, skills and/or structural).

Opportunities might relate to unexploited potential strengths, expected changes, options for career development pathways, and hobbies and interests that might usefully be expanded.

Threats include factors and circumstances that prevent you from achieving your aims for personal, professional and practice development.

Prioritise the most important factors, and draw up goals and a timed action plan.

9 Compare your performance (*see* Module 13 on Accountability and performance) with externally set standards in an open learning culture

There are some assessment programmes with externally set criteria and standards. Standards may be relative (i.e. referenced to norms) or absolute (i.e. referenced to criteria). You could compare your performance against external criteria for clinical practice, record keeping, access and availability, dealing with emergencies, professional–patient relationships, and handling mistakes or complaints. Some examples are given below.

The Denplan Excel Accreditation Programme

This is a comprehensive support package for dentists. It was introduced in October 1999 as a pilot programme in which 670 dentists took part on a voluntary basis, and it was the first ever such programme to win the 'approval' of the Patients' Association.

The Good Practice Scheme

This scheme was launched in October 2001 and consists of 96 specific requirements organised around the following ten commitment statements.

1 We aim to provide dental care of consistently good quality for all patients.
2 We only provide care that meets your needs and wishes.
3 We aim to make your treatment as comfortable and convenient as possible.
4 We look after your general health and safety while you are receiving dental care.
5 We follow the British Dental Association's guidelines on infection control.
6 We check for mouth cancer and tell you what we find.
7 We take part in continuing professional development to keep our skills and knowledge up to date.
8 We train all staff in practice-wide work systems, and we review training plans once a year.
9 We welcome feedback and deal promptly with any complaints.
10 Every member of the practice is aware of the need to work safely under General Dental Council guidelines.

It is a practice self-assessment against 96 requirements, 50 of which require some form of documentation (infection control, practice policies, notes of practice meetings, training records, etc.).

The Self-Assessment Manual for Standards (SAMS)

This was published by the Faculty of General Dental Practitioners in 1991. It continues to be widely used by dentists as a useful reference for standards.

Practice visit questionnaires used by PCTs

These provide useful checklists for compliance with, for example, health and safety legislation.

Checklists used for the purpose of approving practices for vocational training

Again, these provide a useful guide to what is required/desirable in a modern practice.

Investors in People

Investors in People celebrated its tenth anniversary in 2001. More than 24 000 organisations are currently recognised as Investors in People. It is estimated that over 24% of the UK workforce are now working with the Investors in People Standard, which is based on four key principles:

1   *commitment* – to invest in people in order to achieve business goals
2   *planning* – how skills, individuals and teams are to be developed in order to achieve these goals
3   *action* – to develop and use the necessary skills in a well-defined and continuing programme that is directly tied to business objectives
4   *evaluating* – outcomes of training and development for individuals' progress towards goals, the value achieved and future needs.

Fellowship of the Faculty of General Dental Practitioners

This assessment process allows participants to measure their practice standards and processes against published criteria. The Faculty describes it as the 'highest accolade designed to be achievable by any committed principal dentist, which requires high standards across many disciplines in patient care. It aims to encourage candidates to measure themselves and their practice against the Fellowship criteria and provide written evidence that they meet (or even exceed) the requirements, which keep up to date with best current practice'.

10 Observation of your practice

Look at the equipment in your practice. Does everyone know how to operate it properly? Have they been shown this or has it always been assumed that they know anyway?

Ask others what they think of your practice, and invite them to give you some feedback. You could offer to repay the favour by offering them the same facility.

11 Reading/reflecting and refining clinical and non-clinical procedures

Try to read articles in professional journals on a regular basis so that it becomes a habit. Many journals now carry summaries of articles, and these are useful for obtaining a quick overview of the topic under discussion. Actively reflect[1] on what the key relevant messages mean for you.

12 Educational appraisal

Discuss your learning needs with trusted friends and colleagues, or approach the local dental tutor or postgraduate dental dean for advice on professional development. It is interesting to note that since April 2002 general medical practitioner principals have been required to take part in appraisal as part of their contract. The intention is to extend this to all other doctors in general practice. In advance of the appraisal discussions, GPs complete questionnaires and compile documentation recording their achievements and challenges during the previous 12 months, and note their future development needs. There is then a full discussion with the appraiser, and the information gathered from the questionnaires acts as a springboard for discussion.

It would not be unreasonable to speculate that a similar system may be introduced for GDPs in time. It already exists in a number of dental organisations and dentists who work within them already participate in the process.

13 Review the business or development plan of your practice

Do you know the contents of all of the official and informal strategic documents that are relevant to your practice? If so, are you aware of the implications for you and your work? Note down any gaps and whether you have any associated learning needs.

Have you discussed business development opportunities with your professional advisers? Are you aware of what grants are currently available or likely to be available in the future? It has been the experience of some health authorities that many practitioners do not apply for the grants and other reimbursements that are available; the reimbursement of business rates for NHS practitioners is just one example. You may want to maintain regular contact with the Local Dental Committee (LDC) or dental adviser to keep abreast of these opportunities.

14 Job appraisal

Good employment practice should include regular job appraisal (e.g. annually). This gives you and your team an opportunity to review how well you/they are doing in relation to your/their job description. Identify your/their learning and training needs and how they may be achieved in the context of your/their current job or by agreed changes to your/their roles and responsibilities.

The principal dentist(s) in the practice may consider peer or partner appraisal with another respected colleague whom you trust and whose opinion you respect.

15 PUNs and DENs

Originally attributed to Dr Richard Eve, GP Tutor in West Somerset, the PUNs and DENs model is a very practical tool.

PUNs stands for *patient's unmet needs* and DENs is an acronym for *doctor's educational needs*. We could adapt the concept to include the team, and list *team educational needs* where it has been identified that a number of team members have similar requirements. It is a form of reflective practice where the clinician should ask the question 'Could I have done anything differently or better?' after treatment or a consultation session with the patient.

PUNs and DENs are non-threatening, learner-centred processes that have been used in general medical practice since 1995.

The advantages[3.1] of this method are as follows.

- It is simple, easy and good fun to use.
- It takes up a minimal amount of time.
- It is relevant to the daily work of general practice.
- It costs you no money and identifies your education and training needs.
- It can help to improve your clinical skills.
- It identifies not only individual needs but also practice needs.

You may want to classify the outcome of your deliberations into the following areas and use the abbreviations as short-hand in any action plan.

- KC = knowledge clinical
- KN = knowledge non-clinical
- S = skill
- A = attitude
- O = organisational.

By doing so, you will be more effective in managing what you need to do.

Reference

1   Greenhalgh T (1997) *How to Read a Paper*. BMJ Publishing, London.

[3.1]Reproduced by kind permission of Dr Richard Eve.

CHAPTER FOUR

The plan: where do you want to be and how do you get there?

Having found out where you are at present, you have to decide where you want to be next before making a plan for clinical governance in your practice. The most practical way to look at this is to think about your aspirations and decide on what you want to happen (this is your destination). Then look at the various ways in which you could bring about these changes. Unlike the space walks discussed in the introduction, this is not rocket science. As with many other things, the chances are that you have this information in your mind already.

Below is an example of how you could provide another footprint of evidence to demonstrate your efforts.

From the practice perspective

Aspiration	Destination example	Route – to your priorities
Practice vision for change	Practice should offer additional services for patients	Training; additional resources; investigate similar models in other practices
	Complete audit cycles regularly	Incorporate principles of clinical audit into regular work; set up regular reviews and time for staff to undertake relevant audits
	Set up and run regular practice meetings	Someone to organise meetings; protected time for the staff to attend
	Improve implementation of evidence-based care in your practice	Training; education; collation of useful resources; clinical meetings; audit and review procedures that are practice based; protected time for discussions with other colleagues in the practice
	Improve the management of complaints	Training for the complaints manager and relevant staff; systematic review of complaints procedures; look at resource material from professional indemnity organisations

continued overleaf

Aspiration	Destination example	Route – to your priorities
Practice vision for change	Monitor standards of support team in clinical and non-clinical areas	Training in review, clinical supervision and systematic audit procedures; rectify substandard practice at individual and team levels; training and education
	Improvement of your stock control system	Standardise materials; review wastage; investigate alternatives; look at use and abuse of materials
	Improvement of access to clinical records	Standardisation of recording of clinical entry data; IT training

Now use the following template to make some notes about some ideas for the future. These will help to shape the vision for your clinical governance plan and your practice.

From the practice perspective		
Aspiration	Destination	Route – to your priorities
Your vision for change		

CHAPTER FIVE

Setting your priorities for developing clinical governance

You will now have been able to make a wish list after following the previous stages on assessment. All practices are different, and your priorities may or may not reflect those of your peers. It is better to select those topics that are tied into *your* practice's priorities. It is important to have clear aims and objectives that are achievable within your time and resource constraints. You can use the SMART acronym to help you:

* S – specific
* M – measurable
* A – attainable
* R – relevant
* T – time based.

Collect information from all members of the team and from the patients before you make any decisions on how to progress.

Remember to take external influences into account. The recent introduction of the requirement to undertake clinical audit or peer review[1] over a three-year period may be high on your priority list. (Note that only the first 15 hours will be funded in any three-year period. The first period commenced on 24 May 2001 and expires on 31 March 2004.)

Other factors to consider when ranking topics in order of priority include the following.

* Are the project aims and objectives clearly defined?
* Is the topic important for the patients and the team?
* Is it feasible?
* Is it affordable?
* Will it make enough difference to justify the effort?
* Does it fit in with other priorities?

You will also need to relate the priorities to your business planning priorities. One of the misconceptions about clinical governance is that it will in some way detract from your business objectives. In fact, the relationship between the two is synergistic.

When you start thinking about it, the chances are that you will have far more ideas than can possibly be implemented.

Remember the highest priority – the service is for the patients who use it or who will do so in the future. It is no different to the core principle of business management – remember that 'the client is king' and that 'all first-rank professional service firms... are organised in small groups around the customer'.[2]

Who should decide which of the topics on your lists of aspirations should be prioritised? The decision has to be representative and not autocratic or idiosyncratic. Look back at the 'routes and branches' model of clinical governance. You will need people to represent each root, trunk and branch. Remember to involve and engage the team and to give them ownership of the concept.

Set dates for completion of the various stages. How will you set standards and evaluate what you have done? You might want to use a table, as for example in Table 5.1 below, which is an adaptation of a Gantt chart, commonly used in business for project management.

Table 5.1   Example of a Gantt chart

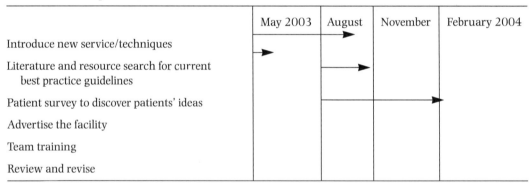

	May 2003	August	November	February 2004
Introduce new service/techniques				
Literature and resource search for current best practice guidelines				
Patient survey to discover patients' ideas				
Advertise the facility				
Team training				
Review and revise				

References

1 Amendment 87, Statement of Dental Remuneration.

2 Peters T (1992) *Liberation Management*. MacMillan, London.

Template for your practice-based clinical governance plan
Photocopy the four pages and complete one chart per priority topic

The topic:
Who chose it?
How was the choice made?

Justify why the topic is a priority:
a personal/practice priority?
a patient priority?
a local/national priority?

Who will be included in the plan?

Who will collect the baseline information and how?

continued overleaf

Where are you now? (baseline)

What information will you obtain about individual learning wishes and needs?
(How will you obtain this and who will do it? Self-completion checklists, discussion, appraisal, patient feedback?)

How will you prioritise everyone's needs in a fair and open way?

Patient input to your plan

continued opposite

Action plan (include objectives, timetabled action, expected outcomes)

How does your clinical governance plan tie in with your other strategic plans for the practice? (e.g. your business development plan)

What additional resources will you require to execute your plan and from where do you hope to obtain them? (Will staff have to pay any course fees or undertake learning in their own time?)

continued overleaf

How much protected time will you allocate to staff to undertake the learning and training described in your plan?

How will you evaluate your learning plan? (Who will be responsible for what?)

How will you know when you have achieved your objectives? (How will you measure success?)

How will you handle new learning requirements as they crop up?

CHAPTER SIX

You have identified your learning needs: what happens now?

A modular approach

As part of a healthcare profession, dentists want to provide high-quality, patient-centred care. This approach is also consistent with good business management of the dental practice. Most of what we need to know follows on here.

The material has been arranged as a series of individual modules. Each module has been prepared to reflect one of the 14 themes of clinical governance.

At the beginning

At the beginning of each module is an introduction to the subject. You might want to pick one or two topics from each of the 14 modules, or work through all of the topics of any single module. You may want to focus on your Terms of Service requirements and do only what is required at the present time from a regulatory point of view, or you may want to tackle the big picture.

The type and number of topics or modules that you choose will depend on what learning needs you have identified from the work you have done up to this point. They will depend on whether you are using this programme to devise your own personal or professional development plan, or are working as a practice team on one or more agreed priority areas, or whether you want to use the material to develop your practice in other ways.

At the end

At the end of each module is:

* a personal learning record for you to complete

- an action plan in which to describe how you will meet your learning needs with respect to the module
- an evaluation chart to record what has been achieved and what education and work are still outstanding.

These record charts have been drawn up in such a way that you can complete them from your own individual perspective, or as a team, or from a practice perspective. Those who have worked with these charts have found them easy to use, and found that they encouraged them to adopt a more structured approach to learning and development. They are part of the footprint of clinical governance.

Use the same tools to evaluate your progress as you used to identify your learning needs – refer back to the variety of methods described earlier in the book.

CHAPTER SEVEN

Baseline review

Your practice

Start collecting evidence about structures, processes and activities in the practice that show you are taking clinical governance seriously. The chances are that you will have a lot of this information in your head already or scattered around the practice. Now it is time to think about collating it and creating a portfolio of evidence that will underpin your clinical governance efforts. Remember that many of your practice management processes can contribute to your portfolio of evidence. For example, your policy on accommodating on-the-day emergencies would provide a good example of how you manage your resources, and can also link into the principles of a patient-centred service.

Clinical governance is essentially about asking two key questions.

1   Are we practising safely?
2   Is what we do effective?[1]

1   Structures

- Dental records – paper or electronic – can you demonstrate whether they are accurate, comprehensive, with updated medical histories? What are the access arrangements and how secure are they? Is confidentiality protected? Are radiographs stored appropriately and are they easily accessible? (Or do you have to sift through dozens of small white envelopes looking for the right ones?)
- Computer system and its capability – is it set up for routine searches of patient data?
- Equipment – collate the instructions for use and maintenance, repair and servicing history. You could do this on a surgery-by-surgery basis and keep a folder in each operating room, or hold the information on computer.

2   Leadership

- Who takes the lead on clinical governance? If you have a practice manager, how does their role interface with the responsibilities of other members of the team?

3 Baseline assessment of current performance

- You will be using a variety of the methods described in this book to demonstrate your current performance in a range of key priority areas, with associated action plans for improvement. You may not have written these down, but they provide another footprint of clinical governance.
- Your educational activities – records have to be maintained for a number of reasons. For example, the GDC may request evidence of your continuing professional development activities, or the Faculty of General Dental Practitioners (FGDP) may request confirmation of your attendance at postgraduate meetings. If you are involved in dental vocational training, you will be asked to demonstrate your commitment to postgraduate education each time you apply to participate in a vocational training scheme.

4 Action plan for developing clinical governance

- Use the template on pages 37–40 to show how you are addressing clinical governance with a number of timetabled action programmes. These do not have to be radical and innovative, and in reality they will be things you want to develop for your practice anyway. The difference may be that until now you have been carrying the ideas around in your head, and this might be a good time to get them down on paper. Photocopy the four pages of the chart for separate exercises addressing different topics. Involve as many people in the practice as you can – this will share the burden of the work and gain ownership of the programme. Remember that clinical governance is a team effort.

The footprints of evidence

In brief, the evidence should include details of the following:

- the overall approach to clinical governance
- human resources, education, training and development, and appraisal initiatives to support clinical governance
- 'knowledge management', data and information systems to support clinical governance – this will include such issues as confidentiality, record keeping, and access to information
- audit, evidence-based practice, and research and development initiatives to support clinical governance
- complaints, risk management and adverse incident initiatives to support clinical governance

• an annual summary of activities – an annual report if you like, which could include information about your achievements and the opportunities of which you are aware for further development. Note your weaknesses, too, and describe how you are planning to overcome them.

Finally, it is worth keeping up to date with the requirements of the big picture because we need to be sure that the clinical governance culture which is developing is consistent with what is happening across the NHS.[2,3]

It may be helpful to bear a few things in mind. Remember to:

1 establish leadership, accountability and working arrangements
2 conduct a baseline assessment of capacity and capability
3 formulate and agree a development plan in the light of this assessment
4 clarify reporting arrangements for clinical governance in your practice/staff handbook.

References

1 Jiwa M (2001) *Clinical Governance: a new panacea for primary care.* Wisdom Centre, Sheffield.

2 Department of Health (1999) *Clinical Governance: quality in the new NHS.* Department of Health, London.

3 van Zwanenberg T and Harrison J (eds) (2000) *Clinical Governance in Primary Care.* Radcliffe Medical Press, Oxford.

PART TWO

The 14 themes of clinical governance

This section of the book is arranged in modules. For each module you will find:

- key information about the topic
- who could do what
- your action plan
- your evaluation plan
- your record of learning.

Establishing and sustaining a learning culture

'Clinical indicators should be used to learn, not to judge.'[1] The fact that this needs stating shows how fragile the learning culture of the NHS really is. Medical and dental students were traditionally humiliated if they were unable to come up with the right answer, in front of other students, patients and nursing staff. Clinical audit has sometimes been used to identify and expose people's shortcomings rather than to provide opportunities for learning and improvement.

The recent introduction of league tables of performance is another example of valuable information sometimes being used out of context, concealing the all-important fact that like was not necessarily being compared with like – and you know what they say about statistics.

Clinical governance will only achieve health gains and improvements in the quality of healthcare if team members are not penalised for admitting mistakes and calling for more resources. Such a culture would help everyone, professionals and managers alike, to work together to achieve the highest standards of care.

Establishing a learning culture that underpins clinical governance

An environment in which clinical effectiveness can flourish requires clinicians and the support team to work together as a team and to involve patients in the process.

The application of clinical governance in practice will require a learning culture that encourages a sustained quality improvement culture, motivated staff and an evaluation of changes in practice. This culture already exists in many dental practices, but it may not be visible to the outside observer. Clinical governance helps to create that visibility.

The components of clinical governance are already established concepts whose roots are based in a learning culture:

- high standards – of care and service provision
- reflective practice – learning from experience
- risk management – of clinical and organisational matters
- personal and team development.

As clinical governance is about delivering uniformly good care as a co-ordinated team, the learning opportunities should involve the team. The education and training plan for the team should address service issues and individuals' development; the strategy should focus on ways of implementing the education and development plan and overcoming barriers to its application.

These barriers, which are common to most healthcare professionals, have been identified as follows:[2]

- isolation of health professionals, even many of those who appear to work in a team
- 'tribalism' as different disciplines protect their traditional roles and responsibilities
- lack of incentives to take up learner-centred, interactive education as opposed to more passive modes of educational delivery (postgraduate qualifications are one example where the uptake of some examinations has been disappointingly low because of a perceived lack of incentives)
- differing rights to time and funds for continuing education between different members of the team within the same practice
- practitioners overwhelmed by the workload and having little time for continuing education
- dissonance between what individuals think they need to learn and what is relevant to real-world needs
- reluctance to develop or accept new models of working
- fear of and resistance to change.

Experienced practitioners will have encountered many of these in the day-to-day running of their practices.

Drawing up educational programmes for your practice

A number of dentists regularly receive training in educational theory and practice of work-based training through their involvement in dental vocational training schemes. The principles of vocational training are common to all work-based learning and include:

- learning *for* work
- learning *at* work
- learning *from* work.[3]

Individuals' own educational plans should complement and dovetail into the overall business and development plans for the practice.

At one recent workshop and seminar on clinical governance, the delegates were asked about their approach to continuing education and training for staff. It was found that 80% did not have any such plans in place. Of the remaining 20%, the vast majority used in-practice resources but did not formally record the activities that took place. A small number had experience of the processes through their recent involvement with vocational training schemes.[4]

Making your own personal learning plan

Your plan should encompass the context and culture of your working environment as well as the knowledge and skills relevant to general dental practice. Your personal learning plan might also form the major part of a future professional revalidation programme. Your plan should:

- identify your weaknesses in knowledge, skills or attitudes
- specify topics for learning as a result of changes in your role, responsibilities or the organisation
- describe how you identified your learning needs
- prioritise and set your learning needs and associated goals
- justify your selection of learning goals
- describe how you will achieve your goals and over what time period
- describe how you will evaluate learning outcomes.

Appropriate mode of delivery

People choose to learn in ways that they are used to, or which are most convenient, rather than the most appropriate method for the topic they need to learn about.

A recent survey of education and training needs showed how health professionals and managers opted for the mode of training with which they were most familiar (usually a lecture or validated professional course) or which suited their working conditions. Few matched their educational requirements with the mode of delivery that was most appropriate for the topic, because commercial and business factors come into play.

Lectures are only useful for transferring knowledge. If active discussion is an essential part of learning, then you would be better joining in small group work and interactive discussion. Most of the new concepts of training for dentists require a change of focus away from didactic methods towards interactive peer group discussions where views and experiences can be shared. The lecture format has been shown to be a motivational and inspirational tool rather than an effective educational strategy.[5]

Problem solving and thinking is an effective approach to learning, and is now widely used in vocational training programmes. The seven stages are as follows.

1   Clarify terms and concepts in the problem.
2   Define the problem – set out what needs to be understood.

3   Analyse the problem – generate possible explanations.
4   Make a systematic inventory of the explanations – link ideas.
5   Formulate learning questions – what you need to be able to understand.
6   Collect information – try to find the answers.
7   Synthesise and test the information – test your answers and discuss the findings.

Learning about such complex subjects as clinical governance or teamworking involves the following:

•   cultural change
•   flexibility to adapt to new roles and responsibilities
•   negotiation and political awareness.

Education about the meaning of clinical governance could be delivered using a range of resources, such as:

•   paper-based activities
•   e-learning
•   workshops
•   lectures, seminars and tutorials.

This format has been described as the concept of blended learning,[6] and is currently being piloted as an Internet-based initiative by the e-learning team at smile-on.com.

This combination approach has been used by a number of primary care trusts/strategic health authorities.

Any such activities should be as interactive as possible to encourage a deeper under-standing of the issues, and of the consequences of action or omission. People learn in different ways, so there should be a variety of methods of education and training on offer so that individuals can opt for the methods they prefer, by which they are more readily engaged and learn best.

Multiprofessional education

Multiprofessional education and training for the NHS workforce is envisaged as being integral to delivering the programme of modernisation of the NHS.[7] There are limited opportunities for GDPs to become involved in multidisciplinary training. The reasons for this are included in the following list of perceived barriers to multiprofessional shared learning:[8]

•   a lack of time – often used by dentists as an excuse for not attending local meetings
•   the medical model inhibiting 'multiperspective communication' – dentists sometimes feel that medical models are adapted for dental practice and are not always entirely appropriate
•   organisational structures and processes – making collaborative practice difficult to maintain

- mistaken assumptions about the meaning of multiprofessional learning being about topics that are common to everyone, rather than being about the different professions contributing to a co-ordinated team.

Continuing professional development and lifelong learning

Continuing professional development (CPD) has been defined as 'a process of lifelong learning for all individuals and teams which enables professionals to expand and fulfil their potential and meets the needs of patients and delivers the health and healthcare priorities of the NHS'.[9]

The principles of CPD apply to non-clinical staff just as much as to clinicians, although there is no formal monitoring of CPD for the professions complementary to dentistry.

CPD is concerned with the following:

- pursuing personal and professional growth by widening, developing and changing your own roles and responsibilities
- keeping abreast of and accommodating clinical, organisational and social changes that affect professional roles in general
- acquiring and refining the skills needed for new roles or responsibilities or career development
- putting individual development and learning needs into a team and multiprofessional context.[10]

Criteria for successful learning[11]

The most successful continuing professional development involves learning which:

- is based on what is already familiar to the learner
- is led by the learner's own identified needs
- is problem-centred
- involves active participation by the learner
- uses the learner's own resources – built on their previous experiences
- includes relevant and timely feedback
- is given when the learner experiences the need to know something
- includes an element of self-assessment.

Lifelong learning combines formal and informal learning as a natural part of everyone's everyday lives.

Evidence-based education
(*see* Module 5 on Evidence-based practice and policy)

Evidence-based education is as important as evidence-based health policy, practice or management. Obtain and read complete papers rather than relying on interesting-looking abstracts. Then make up your own mind about the reliability of the evidence as applied to your own situation.

You could apply evidence-based education in your workplace tomorrow in teaching patients, or by applying to become a trainer on a vocational training scheme, or by offering your experience to facilitate the development of less experienced colleagues.

References

1   Mulley A (1999) Learning from differences within the NHS. *BMJ*. **319**: 528–30.

2   Chief Nursing Officer (1998) *Integrating Theory and Practice in Nursing*. NHS Executive, London.

3   Seagraves L, Osborne N, Neal P *et al.* (1996) *Learning in Smaller Companies (LISC) Final Report*. University of Stirling, Stirling.

4   Rattan R (2001) *Taking the Plunge – clinical governance*. Seminar evaluation (data on file). Croydon PCT, London.

5   Rattan R (1998) *The Lecture: education vs performance*. Dissertation. LPMDE, London.

6   Noam Tamir, CEO smile-on.com. Personal communication (2002).

7   National Health Service Executive (1998) *Working Together. Securing a quality workforce for the NHS*. Department of Health, London.

8   Miller C, Ross N and Freeman M (1999) *Researching Professional Education*. Research Reports Series No 14. English National Board for Nursing, Midwifery and Health Visiting, Cambridge.

9   Calman K (1998) *A Review of Continuing Professional Development in General Practice*. Chief Medical Officer, Department of Health, London.

10   Standing Committee on Postgraduate Medical and Dental Education (SCOPME) (1998) *Continuing Professional Development for Doctors and Dentists*. SCOPME, London.

11   Roland M, Holden J and Campbell S (1999) *Quality Assessment for General Practice: supporting clinical governance in primary care groups*. National Primary Care Research and Development Centre, University of Manchester, Manchester.

Pro forma for assessing whether topic of learning is a priority

Check out whether a particular topic (for anyone in the team) is a priority and whether the way in which the learning will take place is appropriate. Photocopy this pro forma for future use.

> **The topic:**

How have you identified your learning need(s)?

a	Clinical requirement ❏	e Appraisal need ❏
b	Practice business plan ❏	f New to post ❏
c	Legal mandatory requirement ❏	g Individual decision ❏
d	Job requirement ❏	h Patient feedback ❏
		i Other ❏

....

Have you discussed or planned your learning needs with anyone else?

Yes ❏   No ❏   If so, who? ....

What are the learning need(s) and/or objective(s) in terms of:

Knowledge. What new information do you hope to gain to help you to do this?

....

Skills. What should you be able to do differently as a result of undertaking this development?

....

Behaviour/professional practice. How will this impact on the way in which you then do things?

....

Details and date of desired development activity:

....

Details of any previous training and/or experience you have in this area/dates:

....

Your current performance in this area compared with the requirements of your job:

Need significant development in this area	❏	Need some development in this area	❏
Satisfactory in this area	❏	Do well in this area	❏

Level of relevance to practice this area has with regard to your role and responsibilities:

Has no relevance	❏	Has some relevance	❏
Relevant	❏	Very relevant	❏
Essential	❏		

Describe what aspect of your job, and how the proposed education/training, is relevant:

....

Do you need additional support in identifying a suitable development activity?

Yes ❑   No ❑

What do you need?

Describe the differences or improvements for you and the practice:

....

Determine the level of priority of your proposed educational/training activity:

Urgent ❑   High ❑   Medium ❑   Low ❑

Describe how the proposed activity will meet your learning needs rather than any other type of course or training on the topic:

....

If you had a free choice, would you want to learn this? Yes/No

If **no**, why not? (please circle all that apply):

Waste of time
Already done it
Not relevant to my work or career goals
Other

If **yes**, what reasons are most important to you? (put them in rank order):

Improve my performance
Increase my knowledge and understanding
Help me with a further or higher qualification
Just interested
Be better than my colleagues
Do a more interesting job
Be more confident
It will help me
Self-satisfaction
Income generation/another income source

Some ideas on who could do what to establish a learning culture in your practice

The GDP

- Give a lead on the importance of education for all staff.
- Take responsibility for good employer practices for your team.
- Provide adequate resources for all staff to have sufficient opportunities for learning and development.
- Draw up, carry out and evaluate your own professional development plan.

The practice manager

- Organise and review the practice-based professional development plan.
- Obtain facts and figures, and subjective and objective data about learning needs to inform the practice-based plan.
- Encourage individuals to formulate and implement professional development plans.
- Undertake job appraisals for all staff; clarify learning needs and plan to address those needs.
- Identify suitable educational events and activities for staff.
- Recognise staff learning needs associated with clinical governance.

The dental nurse

- Draw up, carry out and evaluate own professional development plan.
- Contribute to teaching/advising patients about oral health and practice services.
- Learn more about applying clinical governance in everyday practice.

The receptionist

- Draw up, carry out and evaluate own professional development plan.
- Arrange and organise in-house educational meetings as requested.
- Help practice manager to obtain baseline data on performance to help to formulate practice-based plan and clinical governance programme.
- Pass on suggestions and comments from patients to practice manager that might serve to identify learning needs of the practice team.

Action plan. Module 1: learning culture

Today's date: ....   Action plan to be completed by: ....

Tackled by	Identify need/assess problem	Plan of action: what will you do?/by when?
Individual – you		
Practice team – you and your colleagues		
Organisation – your practice		

Evaluation: learning culture

Complete an evaluation of progress by ....

Level of evaluation: perspective or work done on this component by	The need or problem	Outcome: what have you achieved?	Who was involved in doing it?	Evaluated: • by whom? • when? • what method was used?
Individual – you				
Practice team – you and your colleagues				
Organisation – your practice				

Record of your learning about 'a learning culture'

Write in topic, date, time spent and type of learning activity

	Activity 1	Activity 2	Activity 3	Activity 4
In-house formal learning				
External courses				
Informal and personal				
Qualifications and/or experience gained				

Managing resources and services

Dental practices run on two types of fuel – people and things.

We all know from experience that if we can recruit the right *people*, then the organisation and management of the practice have the potential for excellence in all respects. In a recent survey of vocational trainers with a minimum of 20 years' clinical experience, staff recruitment, training, motivation and loyalty were identified as the most challenging aspects of running a dental practice.

The *things* are the vast array of mechanical and electronic gadgets that enable us to perform clinical dentistry.

General dental practitioners have to be good at the business of dentistry, and many of the aspects of clinical governance relating to the effective management of resources exist in most practices already. They have to because the cost of mismanagement of resources invariably leads to declining profits.

You must also make sure that the things you need are in the right place at the right time and working correctly. This has everything to do with sound practice management, but it is also a feature of clinical governance.

Getting the right person for the job

The job description

The clearer you are about what you need, the more likely you are to recruit well. Draft a job description that describes all of the tasks and responsibilities of the position, together with the minimum qualifications and experience necessary. If you are filling an existing position, ask the outgoing person to record all of the things that are involved and review the list. Now is the time to add or remove any duties or requirements. It is not so easy to do this afterwards.

Where do you look?

- Advertising – use the local and professional press as appropriate.
- Word of mouth – a valuable recruitment tool. Speak to professional colleagues, local company representatives, local vocational training advisers and postgraduate tutors.
- Internal recruitment – this is useful if someone wants to change roles (e.g. from receptionist to manager). The advantage is that the individual is already known, and they know the ethos of the organisation. Training someone whose skills, knowledge and attitudes you already know about may be a more certain way to get what you want than hoping to find the right person from another organisation.
- Temporary employment – this is a good way of 'trying people out' before you employ them long term. Agencies are particularly useful when you need someone urgently or are not sure for how long someone will be needed.
- Internet sites – a number of sites now offer recruitment facilities.

The interview

Use the job description to draw up an interview outline. You need to use this to make sure that you check all of the attributes and skills that you require *and* to show that you did not reject anyone because of bias or prejudice. Draft your questions beforehand, make them relevant to the job description and record all of the answers to the questions. Take plenty of notes or you will not remember who was who.

You need to ask people:

- why they have applied
- what they can do for your organisation
- how they would fit in with the present team of workers
- when they could start
- whether they will come for the money you can afford.

Make sure that you let people know when they can expect an answer to their application. Ensure that your applicant confirms acceptance before notifying the others that they have not succeeded. *Always* check references before offering a job.

View references with caution. For example, you may receive a good one because an employer is glad the person is moving on, but has no firm evidence on which to condemn him or her.

It can be helpful to divide your candidates into those who:

- could do the job
- could do the job with extra training
- are unsuitable.

Make sure that you are not rejecting people in the last category because of their ethnic origin, sex, age, marital status, religion or disability (not only is this illegal, but it may also prevent you getting the best person for the job).

Before the new employee starts

Plan how your new employee will know what to do. They need a period to learn the ropes, preferably guided by someone who knows how to do the jobs on the job description list. You will not get the best out of someone who has to find out everything from scratch. A new employee needs a mentor or a list of useful people to ask.

Employment law

You need to show that you are managing your staff correctly, so make sure that you provide:

•   an up-to-date job description
•   the terms of employment
•   mutual assessment appraisals and individual training and development plans
•   in-house training with other staff
•   regular meetings with other staff and clear methods of communicating with them at other times
•   knowledge of disciplinary and grievance procedures
•   personnel records kept securely with access only to authorised people.

These are all footprints of clinical governance.

Motivating people to do a better job

It is human nature for people to respond better to praise than to punishment (if you need to use the latter approach, look at the sections on when things go wrong (*see* page 67) and ending and termination of employment (*see* page 68). To put it another way, you get more of the behaviour that you reward.

You cannot praise people unless you know what they are meant to be doing – so be aware of their goals and tasks. You do need to be careful not to become caught up in the details of how they achieve their goals, or they will think that you do not trust them to do the job, or that you have not made the transition from worker to manager. It seems simple to decide to reward everyone equally – but is this motivating?

> Miss A completes a job before the time allocated for it and without any errors. Miss B runs over the time, and the work contains several errors. You give Miss A some more work to do while Miss B struggles to complete hers correctly. If you reward Miss A and Miss B equally, Miss A will feel punished and not at all motivated to do so well next time – all she gets is more work! She is being penalised for being efficient.

The best way to discover what motivates people is to ask them. Some will want more money, others more time, some more flexibility in their work schedule, and yet others to do new and more challenging jobs. Observe how each person responds to the rewards you can offer.

Start with the positive and with the small things. Most of us are not making earth-shattering advances every day, but little achievements and completions. The praise should come:

- immediately after the successful completion of part or all of the task
- from someone who knows what the task involved
- from an understanding of what the task involved.

Incentives that work include the following:

- personal or written congratulations from a respected colleague or immediate superior
- public recognition
- announcement of success at team meetings
- recognising that the last job was well done and asking for an opinion of the next one
- providing specific and frequent feedback (positive first)
- providing information about how the task has affected the performance of the organisation or management of a patient
- encouragement to increase their knowledge and skills so that they can do even better
- making time to listen to ideas, complaints or difficulties
- learning from mistakes and making visible changes.

Also remember the old adage that it is better to praise in public but criticise in private.

Working in teams

See Module 8 on Coherent teamwork for a more detailed discussion of the development and evaluation of teams.

Clinical governance requires teamworking at all levels within the organisation. The practice principal(s) need to give effective leadership as well as enabling the correct mix of team members.

Team members need to respect each other's skills and contributions. All members should be clear about their roles and responsibilities. Remember that each team member brings their worries and previous experience to meetings – look out for the hidden agendas beneath the table.

Three dimensional co-ordination and management

Think about managing and co-ordinating in different directions – not only managing and relating to the staff who are responsible to you, but in all directions (*see* Figure M2.1).

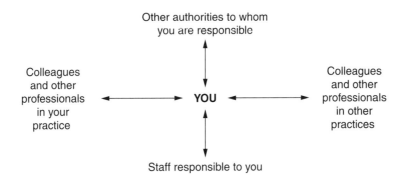

Figure M2.1   Your management responsibility.

Dealing with change

Change happens all the time. The management of the change process is crucial for effective practice development. Think how you can help to make transitions occur smoothly by:

- deciding on what needs to be changed through gathering evidence
- sharing the responsibility for identifying the problem and finding the solutions so that everyone feels part of the process (ownership)
- building in plenty of time to discuss the planned changes so that everyone feels that they have had a chance to put their point of view
- making the changes in small steps
- giving plenty of support and monitoring progress
- giving feedback so that everyone knows how the changes are progressing and what their part in them means to the whole
- celebrating completion and continuing monitoring to prevent backsliding!

Despite the excitement that changes can bring, we tend to resist change. If quality is to be improved, change is inevitable.

Recognise the signs of resistance in yourself and in others if you:

- use outdated methods
- avoid new duties or ways of working
- control and resist the change
- play the victim and use others to do the new work
- wait for someone else to implement the change
- cease being able to do your present work properly.

It is worth thinking about four levels of change.

1   Do we need to do something new?
2   Should we do things differently (i.e. change a system or process)?
3   Should we do something different (i.e. change the purpose)?
4   Do we need to stop doing something (i.e. does any element of the service need to exist at all)?

Dental practices are like weather systems, constantly changing and shifting. If you change one thing, it affects many others. The environment is constantly altering, so the outside influences need constant monitoring. Strategies have to be flexible. People have to be supported in coping with the constant change. Remember to involve them from the outset and to keep them informed and part of the change process. Imposing change breeds resentment and resistance – GDPs know all about that already! Something called clinical governance might be an example; the 1990 Contract is another.

- What makes *you* want to change?
- What are *your* barriers to change?

Setting targets

People react better if they have a direction of travel. Wandering around aimlessly will only make you frustrated and disappointed.

Look at the self-assessment rating charts at the end of each module and think how you could use them to improve quality in a particular area. A SWOT (strengths, weaknesses, opportunities and threats) analysis[1] will help you to plan (*see* Chapter 2 on identifying learning needs). You need to identify what needs doing, whether it can be done, how it can be done, who needs to be involved, when it needs to be done by and how you will know when it is complete.

Remember the KISS principle (keep it simple and short). If you set up too many targets you will not finish any of them, and everyone will become discouraged. Therefore pick just two or three to begin with and aim to complete them before setting new targets.

When things go wrong

Human beings are ... well ... human. We make mistakes. We are all different. We vary in our attitudes. Part of clinical governance involves making individuals accountable for setting, maintaining and monitoring performance standards.

To improve quality assurance, try using a five-step approach as in Table M2.1 below.

Table M2.1 Steps to improve quality assurance

Step	Action	Example/result
1	Use clear quality standards	90% of patients are seen within 15 minutes of their appointment time
2	Monitor to compare performance with standards	An audit report is produced
3	Draw clear lines of authority to take action if performance does not match standards	The practice principal (for example) discusses the problem with the clinical team who undertake to rectify any problems
4	Be clear about the difference between advisory and management functions	The dentist/dental nurse review work methods and procedure times and agree appointment-book control methods with reception staff
5	Encourage performance management by having clear accountability	Individual team members monitor their own time keeping and liaise with reception staff to keep patients advised of any predictable delays

Dealing with poor performance requires better self-discipline, better systems of mentoring and supervision, a belief in continuous professional education, and whistle-blowing responsibility for all without recriminations.

The steps for dealing with unacceptable performance by team members include the following:

- verbal discussion and plans for training or change linked to remedies for the documented/identified deficiency
- written counselling and/or plans for training or change
- warnings about poor performance and/or attitudes (initially verbal, but then written)
- job reallocation to more supervised tasks, or demotion to lesser responsibility
- termination of employment.

Ending and termination of employment

See previous section on 'When things go wrong' for what to do before you get to this stage.

Resignation

Sometimes people leave voluntarily. If you do not know why they are leaving, find out before the reasons affect their successors. You may want to consider an exit interview – this can be helpful because people are generally more open about expressing their views when they know they are about to leave. Such an interview can help to identify difficulties and conflicts of which you may not necessarily have been aware. Make a note to make changes to avoid the same thing happening again. This is good practice management, and it is also clinical governance. Remember the footprint – keep a record of the event in the form of a file note in the employee's file.

Two nurses left a practice in quick succession to take up employment in a neighbourhood practice. An enquiry into the reasons for this revealed an autocratic system of team management that they had found oppressive. No reporting system had been established. The principal owned three other practices and was 'hardly ever there'. Management responsibility had been delegated to an associate with limited relevant experience. The nurses' concerns could not be heard, and all they did was complain to each other about their dissatisfaction. When one of them left to join a neighbouring practice, the other followed because she heard about a second vacancy from her friend and former colleague. Both nurses commented that they now felt 'valued'.

Involuntary retirements

Redundancies do occasionally occur in general practice. Make sure that you follow the correct legal procedures. Termination of employment for serious offences is fortunately rare. Ensure that you follow the correct legal framework. Examples of offences that may merit dismissal include the following:

- breaches of confidence
- violence or abuse
- misuse of drugs
- failure to carry out responsibilities or duties
- theft or fraud.

If you are in any doubt, always contact your professional indemnity organisation for advice.

Timing of termination of employment

Consider the feelings of the person who is leaving, and time the leaving to cause the minimum of embarrassment. Give them time to clear out their belongings and say farewell. Not only does this minimise resentment, but also it gives the remaining staff the feeling that they are being treated as human beings rather than automatons.

Again, seek the advice of your professional indemnity organisation before embarking on action with regard to employment issues. The law is complex – you must have expert advice before acting.

Budgets

In general dental practice, we have to make hard decisions about how to obtain and deliver value for money.[1]

Whenever a new trend, treatment or technology appears, we need to find out:

- whether it is clinically effective
- whether it is cost-effective – whether an existing or rival technology is slightly less effective but cheaper, and would thus be better used as a first choice
- whether investing in that technology will cause harm elsewhere because of a limited budget – whether we will need to cut back on something else in order to introduce it
- how it will affect the way in which the practice is run
- what other resources will be needed to support it
- how much it will be used and by whom
- whether there is scope for extending its use in other surgeries within the practice
- what the likely cost is
- whether it can be offered/provided within the NHS.

Budgets you need include the following:[2]

- staff
- dental materials
- laboratory fees
- equipment
- premises
- repairs and maintenance
- insurance.

Figure M2.2 is a summary of average expenditure expressed as a percentage, which may give you some idea of how you compare with average statistics and may help you to set budgets in the future.

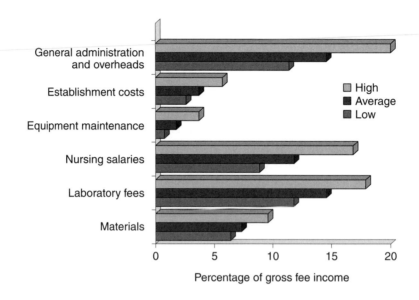

Figure M2.2   Costs (expressed as a percentage of gross fee income) for a range of expenses in a typical dental practice.[3]

Process management

Computerisation is increasingly important for monitoring what is happening in your practice.[4] Maintaining services includes knowing the answers to the following questions.

Who is where?	Draw up a simple grid so that everyone knows where they are working, on what day, and the hours of work. This is particularly important in larger practices, or where a number of part-time staff are employed and where responsibilities are shared
What is where?	Record the items of equipment in each surgery of the practice. This aids accessibility if items are shared, and it also helps with tracking maintenance
Do we have enough?	Stock control – so that you do not run out
When do we need some more?	Track rate of use
When does it need servicing or replacing?	Have a regular routine for this to prevent sudden failure or unexpected expenditure

Delegation

Delegation is about the following:

- authority
- responsibility
- accountability.

One person does not have to do all of this. The structure of general dental practice allows delegation of duties and responsibilities in the following areas:

- clinical areas
- administrative tasks
- managerial functions.

The scope for delegation of clinical duties is limited by legislation in the UK. Dental hygienists are able to undertake periodontal treatment on the dentist's prescription, and dental nurses may be able to take radiographs provided that they have received the appropriate training in this area. At the time of writing, it has just been announced that dental therapists will also be permitted to work in general dental practice.

You may want to consider some of the following areas.

1   Treatment related tasks:

- processing of radiographs
- pouring study casts
- construction of special trays
- fabricating templates and mouthguards (outside the mouth)
- equipment maintenance
- sterilisation
- maintenance of infection control procedures
- patient supervision.

2   Administrative tasks:

- appointment scheduling
- computer record keeping
- fee calculations
- stock control
- patient recall system.

3   Managerial tasks:

- staff management and liaison
- banking
- invoice reconciliation
- schedule checking
- accounts management
- paying suppliers
- PAYE calculation and related activities.

Each person should be given responsibility for their own sphere of activity.
Remember that sometimes simple methods are best.

The practice manager was increasingly frustrated by complaints from the nurses that equipment and materials were disappearing from the surgeries. They sometimes reappeared several days later or were found in another room. Recording showed that a significant amount of time was wasted searching for them. After a practice meeting a procedure was agreed. A book recording the equipment and materials was kept in each treatment room. Each time someone borrowed something they were expected to write down their name and where the item was being taken. When it had been returned, the entry was crossed out. Although the recording system was not always followed, only a few items were not returned. The system was shown to reduce the amount of time that was wasted searching for missing equipment and materials.

Some ideas on who should do what to manage resources and services in your practice

The GDP

- Be clear about what tasks and responsibilities are delegated to the practice manager.
- Demonstrate your commitment to teamwork.
- Offer real support to your team, whatever their role.
- Make sure that you recruit the right team for your style of practice.

The practice manager

- Set up clear lines of accountability for all tasks and responsibilities that are delegated to staff.
- Keep good records about staffing matters and resources, such as equipment logs.
- Be consistently good at managing change. Find ways to overcome other people's reluctance to conform to new situations.
- Know what good recruitment and employment practices are, and apply them consistently.

The dental nurse

- Continually try to improve quality of support.
- Anticipate change.

- Work within your capability – don't agree to undertake tasks for which you are insufficiently trained.
- Organise the equipment and materials in the surgery so that they are safe.
- *See* the list of treatment related tasks identified on page 71.

The receptionist

- Support the practice manager in organising the practice on a day-to-day basis.
- Take pride in the practice.
- *See* the administrative tasks highlighted on page 71.

References

1 Lilley R (1999) *Writing Investment Plans and Health Improvement Programmes.* Radcliffe Medical Press, Oxford.

2 Rattan R (1996) *Making Sense of Dental Practice Management.* Radcliffe Medical Press, Oxford.

3 Data (2002) supplied by Sau-Kee Li, Li & Associates, Poole.

4 Benson T and Neame R (1994) *Healthcare Computing.* Longman Group Ltd, Harlow.

Action plan. Module 2: managing resources and services

Today's date: .... Action plan to be completed by: ....

Tackled by	Identify need/assess problem	Plan of action: what will you do?/by when?
Individual – you		
Practice team – you and your colleagues		
Organisation – your practice		

Evaluation: managing resources and services

Complete an evaluation of progress by ....

Level of evaluation: perspective or work done on this component by	The need or problem	Outcome: what have you achieved?	Who was involved in doing it?	Evaluated: • by whom? • when? • what method was used?
Individual – you				
Practice team – you and your colleagues				
Organisation – your practice				

Record of your learning about 'managing resources and services'

Write in topic, date, time spent and type of learning activity

	Activity 1	Activity 2	Activity 3	Activity 4
In-house formal learning				
External courses				
Informal and personal				
Qualifications and/or experience gained				

MODULE 3

Establishing and disseminating a research and development culture

Developing a research and development culture in primary care should encourage the wider adoption of evidence-based practice by all practitioners. This in turn should lead to increasingly appropriate patient management and more cost-effective prescribing practices.

There is a perception that the gulf between academics and GDPs is as wide as ever. Academics do not always convey their conclusions in ways that enable practitioners to make informed choices about treatment options. It is not uncommon for GDPs to criticise researchers for not studying patients in real-life situations, suggesting that some academics may have lost touch with everyday patient care. The flaws in some research studies may also contribute to a sense of distrust of research results in general.

The Department of Health and the NHS spend nearly £500 million per annum on research. In addition, industry (mainly pharmaceuticals) spends about £2500 million, medical charities spend more than £400 million and the Medical Research Council spends nearly £300 million per annum. Little of this research funding is invested in primary care issues or settings. The intention is that future research and funding will be more in line with NHS priorities and needs and the health of communities, and will encourage networks of research and development activity.

Research in primary care

The 'NHS Research and Development strategy aims to create a knowledge-based health service in which clinical, managerial and policy decisions are based on sound information about research findings and service developments'.[1]

As general practitioners, we are at the coalface of primary care and we may feel that research is someone else's priority. A multidisciplinary approach to primary care research and development is important.[1] Primary care is generally acknowledged to be a vastly under-researched area. Primary care research encompasses epidemiology and the natural history of conditions, the clinical encounter, the patient perspective on care, engagement of the patient in decision making, organisation of the delivery of primary care services, delivery of care across the interfaces of health, management of resources and the implementation of change.

Research and development are essential activities for understanding whether or not care is effective, and how to make the best use of resources. However, there is a considerable gap that needs to be bridged between research findings 'proving' best practice, and GDPs applying those findings in their everyday work. The true benefits of research and development will only be realised when there is a demonstrable impact on patient care from practitioners implementing lessons from research as a routine aspect of their work.

Establishing a research and development culture in your practice

Unless you have an expert in your practice team or you are already part of a research network, it may be better to focus on 'development' than on 'research'. Your approach will include the following:

- understanding how to find out more about the evidence for best practice in investigation, management or treatment in clinical practice or organisational matters
- knowing how to access the findings in published literature and research papers
- creating an infrastructure with access to the evidence – an up-to-date practice library, links to the Internet, and links to other sources of information about the demographic characteristics of the local population
- links to the local postgraduate centre, a nearby dental school, or the local division of the Faculty of General Dental Practitioners (FGDP) to suit your particular areas of interest
- knowing of or arranging skills training in research methods (e.g. questionnaire surveys or focus groups) from your postgraduate centre or the FGDP
- collaborating with others who have more expertise as a way of getting started – identify and enter suitable patients in their studies after you have obtained your patients' informed consent
- holding a journal club in your practice to present and debate interesting and current published papers
- looking for topics that are important in your locality. For example, could you investigate a particular health issue? Is a new model of delivery of care worth piloting? Your PCT may have a view on this. Over the years a number of new initiatives have been piloted at local and national level through the PDS schemes
- thinking about how you might record all contacts with patients in a more systematic way to enable you to undertake research on your practice population more readily
- encouraging the integration of evaluation in all aspects of practice work.

Don't bite off more than you can chew – keep any research work focused on the question and purpose of the study. You may want to consider areas that will benefit your practice as a business as well as improve the quality of patient care. The two objectives do not have to be mutually exclusive.

Critical appraisal

Reading and evaluating a paper is mainly about applying common sense. Critical appraisal is a basic skill that any healthcare professional can readily learn and apply to their own situation. You will soon discover for yourself some of the common flaws in published studies, sometimes even in respected peer-reviewed journals where mistakes were over-looked by the publication team.

In general, you should consider whether:[2,3]

- the paper is relevant to your own practice and the results are applicable to your own circumstances
- the research question is clear and well defined
- any definitions are unambiguous
- the context of the study is described
- the aim(s) and/or objective(s) of the study are clearly stated
- the design and methodology are appropriate for the aim(s) and the question posed
- the measuring instruments seem to be reliable, so that different assessors at different points in time would make the same observations
- the investigator is actually measuring that which they intend to measure
- the sampling method is clear
- the outcomes that are chosen to evaluate any intervention are appropriate
- the results relate to the aim(s) and objective(s) of the study
- the results seem to be robust and justifiable
- there are any biases in the method or the results, such as non-reporting of drop-outs from the study
- any unanticipated outcomes are explained
- the conclusions are valid
- you have any other concerns about the study.

Good practice with questionnaires in general

Questionnaires are often used as the tool of choice for finding out the answer to a particular question. It is a misconception that undertaking a questionnaire survey is one of the simplest and easiest methods. In fact, designing and employing a questionnaire is full of pitfalls, and it is one of the most difficult techniques to use to gain a true or valid answer to the question posed.

Questionnaires are useful for finding out information about the following:

- attitudes
- behaviours
- opinions
- beliefs.

For the results to be valid and accurate, the respondents must be representative of the target population. The response rate should be high and as near to 100% as possible.

Pilot your draft questionnaire on people who will not be included in your final survey. The pilot should detect any problems with your questions or method.

Benefits of a postal questionnaire survey

- It is relatively cheap, as it does not involve interviewers.
- One skilled person can design the project, while less skilled staff undertake data collection.
- It is repeatable.
- It can be distributed over a wide geographical area.
- It can obtain the views of many people, although a large survey is costly.

Drawbacks of a postal questionnaire survey

- It is relatively time-consuming due to chasing up non-respondents and performing analyses.
- Response rates tend to be lower than for interview surveys.
- People who are illiterate, have learning disabilities, are visually impaired or suffer mental health problems, elderly people and those from ethnic minority groups with poor English language skills are unlikely to complete questionnaires.
- One cannot be sure who has answered the questionnaire.
- Respondents may give dishonest answers.
- Respondents cannot clarify a question that they do not fully understand.
- People may give their opinion on topics they know little or nothing about.

A protocol for conducting a patient survey using a self-completion questionnaire

If you decide to undertake a survey of patients' views on an issue (*see* Module 10 on Meaningful patient involvement), write out your protocol first so that you adopt a scientific design and do not make up the method as you go along.[4]

1   Decide on the exact question being posed. Here are some points to bear in mind about questions.

- Avoid double questions – try to make each question focused and include only one idea per question.

- Avoid abbreviations.
- Avoid open-ended questions whenever possible.

2   Decide on your rating scale. You may want to consider some of the following.

- *A Likert-type scale.*[5] Subjects are asked to express their level of agreement or disagreement with a five-point scale. Each level of agreement is given a numerical value from 1 to 5. A statement is made and the subject is asked to mark whether they strongly agree, agree, neither agree nor disagree, disagree or strongly disagree with that statement. The Likert scale has been shown to have a high degree of reliability and validity, and has been demonstrated to be effective for measuring change over a period of time.
- *A semantic Likert scale.* You could use a scale, say, from 1 to 7 where 1 was rated as excellent and 7 was rated as poor.
- *Ranking.* You could include a number of features of your practice and ask patients to rank them in order of priority for them.

3   Write down the purpose or aim of the survey on the questionnaire.
4   Define your target population.
5   Consider the level of resources available to undertake the survey – your own and others' time, expertise in designing questionnaires and coding and analysing data, funds for printing and postage, etc.
6   Write out your protocol, which should include the following:

- the number to be sampled (50–100 is a good sample size)
- the way in which sampling will be carried out
- a description of the pilot phase
- the method of delivery of the questionnaire
- the way in which completed questionnaires will be returned
- how and when non-respondents will be chased up
- the outcomes by which achievement of the purpose will be measured
- the mode of dissemination of results – patient notice or newsletter
- the likely action plan that will result.

7   Find out whether an established and valid questionnaire already exists. One useful example is the *General Practice Assessment Survey*,[6] which measures access and availability, technical care, interpersonal care, continuity of care, trust, contextual knowledge, referral and co-ordination of care outside the practice. It is freely available to use, but will require some modification to adapt it to general dental practice. Carry out preliminary work to gather people's views about the content and purpose of the survey.
8   Adopt the usual wording of your target population – keep the questionnaire reasonably short, and don't include any unnecessary or meaningless questions.
9   Try out the questionnaire on people who will not be included in your sample population. Ask them to give you constructive feedback on your questions. Then refine your questionnaire and method accordingly.

10   Start your survey. Make it easy for respondents to return the questionnaires by sup-
      plying stamped addressed envelopes, a Freepost address, easily accessible collection
      boxes, etc.
11   Remind non-respondents once or twice, depending on your resources, time frame
      and how important it is to have as high a response rate as possible.

Some ideas on who should do what to establish a research and development culture in your practice

The GDP

• Give a lead in establishing research and development in the practice (e.g. make
  resources available or include the topic in your business and development plan).
• Co-operate with any research studies that are being undertaken at the postgraduate
  centre or as part of a Faculty of General Dental Practitioners (FGDP) initiative.
• Apply evidence of best practice to your everyday clinical work.

The practice manager

• Find out what resources are available for conducting a patient survey.
• Map out the expertise and resources for research and development in the practice.
• Apply evidence of best practice to your everyday management role.

The dental nurse

• Co-operate with any research studies based in the practice.
• Apply evidence of best practice to your everyday clinical work.

The receptionist

• Help to collect data for any research studies undertaken in the practice by issuing
  questionnaires and collating responses to them.
• Help to monitor the processes that directly involve patients, and help to explain to
  them the nature of the work that is being undertaken.

References

1   Mant D (1997) *R and D in Primary Care*. NHS Executive, Wetherby.

2   Chambers R (1998) *Clinical Effectiveness Made Easy*. Radcliffe Medical Press, Oxford.

3   Morrison J, Sullivan F, Murray E and Jolly B (1999) Evidence-based education: development of an instrument to critically appraise reports of educational interventions. *Med Educ*. **33**: 890–3.

4   Chambers R (1999) *Involving Patients and the Public: how to do it better.* Radcliffe Medical Press, Oxford.

5   Likert RA (1932) A technique for the the measurement of attitudes. *Arch Psychol*. **140**: 55.

6   National Primary Care Research and Development Centre, University of Manchester; www.npcrdc.man.ac.uk

Action plan. Module 3: establishing and disseminating a research and development culture

Today's date: .... Action plan to be completed by: ....

Tackled by	Identify need/assess problem	Plan of action: what will you do?/by when?
Individual – you		
Practice team – you and your colleagues		
Organisation – your practice		

Evaluation: establishing and disseminating a research and development culture

Complete an evaluation of progress by ....

Level of evaluation: perspective or work done on this component by	The need or problem	Outcome: what have you achieved?	Who was involved in doing it?	Evaluated: • by whom? • when? • what method was used?
Individual – you				
Practice team – you and your colleagues				
Organisation – your practice				

Record of your learning about 'establishing and disseminating a research and development culture'

Write in topic, date, time spent and type of learning activity

	Activity 1	Activity 2	Activity 3	Activity 4
In-house formal learning				
External courses				
Informal and personal				
Qualifications and/or experience gained				

MODULE 4

Reliable and accurate data

Looking at the big picture again, it is sensible to suggest that clinicians, patients and health service administrators need reliable and accurate data to connect individuals or their healthcare records to other knowledge that is relevant to whole patient care.

The purpose of the 'Information for Health' strategy is to help patients to receive the best care and to enable health professionals to provide care and improve the health of the public.

Don't forget that data also need to be confidential (*see* Module 6 on Confidentiality).

The problem in general dental practice is that the quality and availability of useful data are not necessarily all that great unless there are computerised records.

It may be a tongue-in-cheek view, but anecdotal evidence suggests that so far as useful information is concerned, the chances are that Finagle's Laws (from Murphy's stable), apply in that:

1   the information that you have is not the information you want
2   the information that you want is not what you need
3   the information that you need is not available
4   in any collection of data, the figure that is most obviously correct, beyond all need of checking, is probably the one mistake.

On a more serious note, the issue does need to be addressed not only in general dental practice but also in the wider NHS. It is easy to obtain data relating to activity such as waiting times but nearly impossible to get information to monitor clinical quality – and how this may be used to change clinical practice.[1]

Clinical information systems

A clinical information system can be defined 'as one which will contain all the administrative, demographic and person-based information relating to an individual's healthcare which the clinician needs, when and where needed, to provide relevant, evidence-based care to that patient'.[2]

The information available that relates to dentistry is negligible. The Dental Practice Board (DPB) holds statistical data relating to clinical activity, but there are few other examples. Most trusts have systems that have evolved to meet the requirements of contract monitoring, some of which may include information on secondary dental contracts. Given that there is a desire to integrate NHS dentistry with the wider NHS, there will have to be information technology-led initiatives to facilitate this process of integration.

Lifelong electronic health records (EHRs) for everyone

The use of computers to capture, organise and display information has many advantages. It avoids the duplication of data entry, as is illustrated by the following example.

Whilst on holiday, Mr B has been seen at an emergency dental service for the treatment of an acute condition. The dentist at that service has made a note of the condition (first record) and given Mr B a letter to indicate the nature of the problem and to outline the nature of the emergency treatment (second record).

Mr B then attends the practice of his usual dentist, who identifies the need for some restorative work and notes that there have been recurrent episodes of pericoronitis which frequently cause pain, discomfort and swelling for his patient. The usual dentist undertakes the restorative treatment and writes his notes on the patient's record card (third record). He then writes a referral letter to the hospital (fourth record). The appointment clerk at the hospital enters the request (fifth record) and sends an appointment. When Mr B is seen and treated, the oral surgeon makes a clinical record (sixth record) and writes a letter to the referring dentist (seventh record). The letter is added to the patient's bulging file and cannot easily be found at a later date. In the mean time the dentist submits a form (electronic or paper) to the DPB for payment for the work he has carried out (eighth record).

The problems shown by this example are as follows.

- The basic data set of patient details is entered many times over. Time and effort are therefore wasted.
- The clinical data relating to one episode are not all available in one place, but have to be searched for – sometimes without result.
- The opportunity for errors is multiplied each time an entry is made.
- It is difficult, if not impossible, to keep accurate and useful records.

The advantages of electronic health records are as follows.

- They can record the information once.
- They can record the information accurately by using templates or on-screen prompts.
- They can display the information in a variety of ways (e.g. a summary, by treatment item, or a chronological account).

- They can make the information accessible to a variety of people.
- They can make each part of the information subject to different levels of access so that, for example, personal medical information is not available to the non-clinical staff.
- They can supplement information that is not easily available by other means (e.g. how long people have to wait when they attend for their appointment).
- They can be consulted remotely across long distances.

The next example shows what can be done as soon as the necessary equipment is available and data entry is completed. The technology is available to do it now.

Mr W attends as a new patient in London complaining of severe pain and a large facial swelling. He is elderly and confused and lives in Bradford. His daughter does not know the details of his medical history or anything about the recent dental treatment he has undergone. His electronic health record in Bradford is accessed electronically. This shows that he has recently had root canal therapy on a lower second molar. The tooth was non-vital at the time of treatment. He is on anticoagulant therapy and has an allergy to penicillin. The dentist is helped by the record to decide what treatment is best at this stage, and now has an understanding of how the acute dental infection may have arisen.

Secure access at all times to patient records

A paper record has inherent disadvantages.

- It cannot be in two places at once.
- It is difficult to find the information you want in a mass of paper sheets.
- It is inefficient – time is wasted looking for the record, looking through the record and copying out information that is in it.
- It is bulky and difficult to store efficiently.

Make records easy to use so that you:

- minimise the training needed to use them
- prevent security procedures being circumvented
- record or retrieve information at the correct time
- reduce repetitive routine tasks
- enter or retrieve information in a standardised manner
- facilitate communication between all health staff
- incorporate audit and risk management.

The Good European Health Record project was established to develop a common health record architecture, published in the public domain, for Europe.[3]

We have yet to embrace the technology that can make all of this happen. The advantages of smart cards are well documented.[4] They can have different levels of access for different people. For example, a pharmacist could access the medication record but not the results of a patient's chest radiograph, and a dentist could access medical history summaries but not details of unrelated issues. There are financial implications for turning the vision into reality, so the ideal solution may still be some way off.

Information about best practice for GDPs

We all grumble about having to do too much paperwork. Your grumbles may have grown exponentially since you started reading this book. How often have we all read the title of an interesting article or paper and put it to one side with a view to reading it thoroughly later? The fact is that we cannot keep up with the reading that we ought to do. New data gathered in abstract is easily forgotten. What we need is accurate information that is relevant to general practice, accessible at the time when it is needed and applicable to clinical practice.

Vast numbers of papers are published – 20 000 biomedical journals and 17 000 books every year. How much of this information is evidence based? It is impossible for most people to weigh the evidence for every subject about which they need good-quality information.

Information technology can make some contributions.

- Search technology can retrieve abstracts of relevant publications.
- Libraries or user sites can keep you up to date with most of the published data on selected subjects using keywords.
- Best-evidence summaries produced by committees of reviewers are published (*see* Appendix for a list of useful Internet sites).

The National electronic Library for Health (NeLH) should play an increasing role in the organisation, accreditation and updating of clinical reference material, and it will be available on NHSnet. However, it is difficult to see how GDPs will have the time to consult it during working hours! Other members of the team will not only have to find the time but will also need to locate a suitable access point.

The Cochrane Library is another useful resource that is available (*see* Module 5 on Evidence-based practice and policy).

Fast and convenient public access to information and care through online information services

Leaflets, videos and interactive CD-ROMs have all been used by GDPs to promote health, educate patients about treatment options, increase the uptake of necessary treatment, play a part in gaining consent and provide information about specific conditions. The effort that is put into their production does not ensure quality or usefulness. Many of them are an extension of the verbal exhortations given to patients in face-to-face encounters, and some are no more than sophisticated 'selling tools'. Supplying patients with a leaflet or video to back up information has been shown to increase their understanding and knowledge[5] compared with just giving information verbally, but there is scant evidence of associated behaviour change.

Internet sites on health-related topics are myriad. Many of them are of doubtful value and some are positively misleading, but some make a valuable contribution to helping patients to make sense of the many facets of modern dental care.

Discern[6] is a project based at Oxford University to develop a system whereby the public can check the quality of online health information. Another site to help people to assess the quality of information is the Centre for Health Information Quality.[7]

Teledentistry

Teledentistry is the transmission of dental data, including radiographic and photographic images, from one place to another. Healthcare is being changed dramatically by the marriage of computers and telecommunications.[8]

There are concerns about the referral mechanisms that currently operate. In one study,[9] 48% of respondents were not satisfied overall with the service of their current specialist oral surgery referral site. The principal reason given was the length of the waiting time for consultation and treatment.

The electronic transfer of radiographs was theoretically possible at the time when X-rays were discovered. In 1920, transmission of the first dental radiograph was performed by telegraph. Since then, different transmission protocols have been used, including telephone lines and the file transfer protocol through the Internet.

Today, computers are central to image acquisition, processing, enhancement, measurement, storage and retrieval.

The advantages of teledentistry are as follows:

* improved access to specialists to accelerate diagnosis and treatment
* reduced cost of achieving oral health as a result of shared resources
* lessens isolation of practitioners by providing peer support and specialist contact.

Pilot studies to help to overcome the distances that patients might have to travel and the long waiting times for specialist opinions have used remote cameras, imaging or communication programmes. The patient is in a rural dentist's surgery, and the specialist in a central hospital gives an opinion. Such networks may also be used for inter-institutional collaboration and distance learning.

To respond proactively to the digital transformation of oral healthcare, dentists must become familiar with its technologies and concepts. They must learn what new information technology can do for them and their patients, and then develop creative applications that promote the profession and their approaches to care.[8]

Many of the early trials have focused on cases where an orthodontic assessment was required.[10]

Perhaps there will be a future when all patients will consult their health professionals in this way.

Ethical and legal considerations[3]

The purposes of patient records are as follows:

- to benefit the patient by providing a record of care that supports the clinician in the present and the future
- to provide a medico-legal record to support and demonstrate the competence of the clinician
- to keep a contemporaneous note of the clinical condition and treatment provision.

Any other use must be legitimate and implies that consent should be sought. It may include the generation of data for health service management or public health. The process of data aggregation for audit or other quality assurance programmes takes individual clinical record entries out of their original context. Misinterpretation or breaches of confidentiality may occur.

Some data collection can be misleading or faulty because the way in which the data are collected takes no account of clinical procedures. Decisions based on such data will almost always be wrong!

Sharing of information between GDPs and other healthcare professionals to provide seamless care

Increasingly, patients receive their care from 'teams' rather than individuals. With dental access centres now open, there is an increased likelihood that some patients (perhaps only a minority) may receive dental care not only on different occasions but also at different sites. Without the efficient sharing of information, duplication of effort or even harm may result. Ethical and legally acceptable multidisciplinary access to patient information improves care.

Problems can arise if two sets of records – one that the patient holds and one that the professional keeps – have to be completed. One or the other will be neglected unless procedures for duplication of entries are streamlined and simple.

All health professionals need to think of ways in which patient-held records could be produced more simply.

With increasing computerisation of records, it should be possible to give the patient a print-out of the information that they would like to have. This would save time, prevent duplication, and increase autonomy and self-management. A smart card with variable levels of access determined by the patient would be even better!

Some ideas on who should do what to create reliable and accurate data in your practice

The GDP

- Take ultimate responsibility for the security and standard of record keeping.
- Improve the reliability and accuracy of data recording in the practice by checking that there are efficient practices and procedures.
- Provide training for staff so that entries are made when, for example, a patient telephones with a query or to cancel an appointment.
- Obtain guidance on 'good record keeping' from your indemnity provider.

The practice manager

- Devise and organise systems to reduce duplication of data recording.
- Manage the computer system so that it is effective and offers health professionals ready access to patients' records.
- Identify staff learning needs with respect to IT, and organise training as appropriate.

The dental nurse

- Be consistent in keeping accurate records for all of the patients in your care.
- Maintain a record of laboratory work in/out.

The receptionist

- Take care to maintain confidentiality when handling patients' records.
- Be meticulous about entering data in the right records at the right time.

The hygienist

- Access dental records in practice on a 'need-to-know' basis.
- Agree a protocol for recording information relating to this aspect of care.
- Be sure that you work to a prescription from a dentist.

References

1   Lugon M and Scally G (2001) *Clinical Governance Bulletin.* **2**(2). RSM Press, London.

2   The Welsh Office (1999) *Better Information – Better Health. Information management and technology for health care and health improvement in Wales.* The Welsh Office, Cardiff.

3   Griffith SM, Kaira D, Lloyd D *et al.* (1995) A portable communicative architecture for electronic healthcare records: the Good European Health Record project. *Medinfo.* **8**: 223–36.

4   Neame R (1997) Smart cards – the key to trustworthy health information systems. *BMJ.* **314**: 573–7.

5   Coulter A (1998) Evidence-based patient information is important, so there needs to be a national strategy to ensure it. *BMJ.* **317**: 225–6.

6   http://www.discern.org.uk

7   http://www.hfht.org.chiq

8   Bauer J and Brown W (2001) Transformation of oral health care: teledentistry and electronic commerce. *J Am Dent Assoc.* **132**(2): 204–9.

9   Brickley M (2000) Oral surgery – the referral system and teledentistry. *Br Dent J.* **188**: 388–91.

10 http://www.cticm.bris.ac.uk/teledent/Examples.htm

Further reading

Gillies A (1999) *Information and IT for Primary Care.* Radcliffe Medical Press, Oxford.

Kiley R (1999) *Medical Information on the Internet* (2e). Churchill Livingstone, London. (Includes free CD-ROM.)

Tyrrell S (2002) *Using the Internet in Healthcare* (2e). Radcliffe Medical Press, Oxford.

Action plan. Module 4: reliable and accurate data

Today's date: ....   Action plan to be completed by: ....

Tackled by	Identify need/assess problem	Plan of action: what will you do?/by when?
Individual – you		
Practice team – you and your colleagues		
Organisation – your practice		

Evaluation: reliable and accurate data

Complete an evaluation of progress by ....

Level of evaluation: perspective or work done on this component by	The need or problem	Outcome: what have you achieved?	Who was involved in doing it?	Evaluated: • by whom? • when? • what method was used?
Individual – you				
Practice team – you and your colleagues				
Organisation – your practice				

Record of your learning about 'reliable and accurate data'

Write in topic, date, time spent and type of learning activity

	Activity 1	Activity 2	Activity 3	Activity 4
In-house formal learning				
External courses				
Informal and personal				
Qualifications and/or experience gained				

MODULE 5

Evidence-based practice and policy

Incorporating research-based evidence into everyday practice should promote effective working and improve quality. The evidence-based approach is a bridge between science and clinical practice. The dentist must integrate the evidence in the literature with patient preferences, scientific knowledge, clinical judgement and personal experience.[1] The clinical governance culture is all about seeking ways to adopt proven effective practices and replace those that are less effective or more costly.

We need to ask some important questions.

1 Are we doing things in the right way?
2 What is the evidence relating to our practice?
3 How can we ensure that the necessary changes are put into clinical practice?
4 How do we know that the changes made are being sustained?

Definitions

Effectiveness is the extent to which a treatment or other healthcare intervention achieves a desired effect. 'To be reasonably certain that an intervention has produced health benefits it needs to be shown to be capable of producing worthwhile benefits (efficacy and cost-effectiveness) and that it has produced that benefit in practice.'[2] It is important to be clear about the terminology used in relation to evidence-based practice.

Evidence-based care is the 'conscientious, explicit and judicious use of current best evidence in making decisions about the care of individual patients (which means) integrating individual clinical expertise with the best available external clinical evidence from systematic research. This should be done in consultation with the patient in order to decide upon the option which suits that patient best.'[3]

Effectiveness is the extent to which a clinical intervention, procedure, regimen or service, when deployed in the field, does what it is intended to do for a defined population.

Efficacy is the extent to which a specific intervention, procedure, regimen or service produces a beneficial result under ideal conditions.

Gathering the evidence

The development of new techniques and materials in dentistry relies heavily on research. It has been described as 'the major energy source for fuelling professional change' and 'is the very scaffolding on which we build and sustain a practice'.[4] That 'scaffolding' is part of the 'framework' of clinical governance. There are many forms of dental research, ranging from laboratory experiments to case studies and reports, and evidence is available from a number of sources. However, not all of these sources carry equal authority. There is a hierarchy of evidence as shown below, with the most rigorous sources listed first:

1   evidence from systematic reviews of multiple, well-designed, randomised controlled trials
2   evidence from at least one properly designed, randomised controlled trial of appropriate size
3   evidence from well-designed, non-randomised trials, non-controlled intervention studies, cohort studies, time series or case–control studies
4   evidence from well-designed, non-experimental studies from more than one centre or research group
5   opinions of respected authorities based on clinical experience, descriptive studies and reports of expert committees.

(Interestingly, much of what is done in clinical practice is underpinned by what is deemed to be the lowest level of evidence in this hierarchy.)

Where to find it?

There is a view that much research is unwieldy, disorganised and biased, and that much of it is also insufficiently relevant to be clinically useful.[5]

It has been suggested that there are three levels of information.[6]

- *Level 1 information* – this is information that is part of everyday living. Comments such as 'this works better' and 'it looks more natural' are examples, and this vocabulary is used on an everyday basis with patients.
- *Level 2 information* – this may have a scientific basis, but the studies are not in the public domain. There may be references to 'data on file', but this may reflect opinions that may not have scientific credibility.
- *Level 3 information* – this is the source material. It may be a published and refereed paper in a scientific journal. It should provide the basis for clinical decision making.

The resources available to GDPs include the following:

- journals which contain reviews of evidence, such as *Evidence-Based Dentistry*
- the Cochrane Library – available both on CD-ROM and on the World Wide Web
- the NHS Centre for Reviews and Dissemination, University of York
- specialist electronic databases such as Medline.

Systematic reviews of evidence (the term encompasses all attempts to synthesise conclusions from two or more publications on a given subject) are particularly useful for GDPs because they provide a balanced view from a number of studies. They represent an excellent starting point for answering clinical questions.

The NHS Centre for Reviews and Dissemination is a facility commissioned by the NHS Research and Development programme to undertake, commission and identify reviews on the effectiveness and cost-effectiveness of health interventions and disseminate them to the NHS. It produces the following:

- Database of Abstracts of Reviews of Effectiveness (DARE)
- NHS Economic Evaluation Database
- *Effective Health Care* bulletins
- *Effectiveness Matters* – bulletins containing short summaries of systematic reviews with important messages.

As an example, one particularly useful effectiveness bulletin involved the systematic review of 652 relevant papers, of which 253 papers (representing 195 studies) contained the minimum core of data for inclusion in the paper that looked at best practice in dental restorations.[7] Research of this type is particularly useful for busy GDPs, as it contains relevant and practical information, although it must be said that the content in terms of relevance to general dental practice is somewhat limited.

Getting evidence into practice

'Unless research-based evidence and guidance is incorporated into practice, efforts to improve the quality of care will be wasted. Implementing evidence may require health professionals to change long-held patterns of behaviour.'[8]

To bring about a change and get evidence into practice:[8]

- consider what individual beliefs, attitudes and knowledge influence the behaviour of professionals and managers
- be aware of important influences in the organisational, economic and community environments of practitioners
- identify the factors that are likely to influence the proposed change
- plan appropriate interventions: 'multi-faceted interventions targeting different barriers to change are more likely to be effective in achieving change than single interventions'[8]
- keep people informed by describing the evidence and the need for change in words and ways that they can comprehend
- motivate people to tackle the change – show why the change is necessary and important, who else supports the change, and how problems associated with the proposed change can be solved
- provide adequate resources to underpin strategies to change practice (e.g. people to promote that change who have the right level of knowledge and skills)

- incorporate monitoring and evaluation of the change from the planning stage and throughout the activity
- implement the change and find ways to maintain and reinforce the new practices (e.g. reminder systems, educational outreach programmes)
- disseminate information about the change in ways that are appropriate to the nature and setting of the participants.

The implementation of evidence in practice is a complex issue and there are no 'magic bullets'.[9] It has been recognised that the evidence-based movement in dentistry is still in its infancy.[10]

With evidence-based care, patients can be treated differently depending on their risk category. For example, patients who are high risk and caries prone may be offered a more intensive prevention programme involving the use of topical fluoride, chlorhexidine rinses and dietary advice. The result of evidence-based dentistry has been a move away from invasive options and towards prevention in these situations.

In December 1998, JW Robbins wrote that 'with regard to dentistry, these are indeed the best of times ... we can predictably replace missing teeth with implant-supported prostheses ... we can provide more precise surgical and restorative therapy with the aid of improved magnification and illumination ... we can restore missing tooth structure with restorations so natural in feel and appearance that they defy detection.' He went on to say that 'as a profession we have become so enamoured with our new technologies that we seem to have lost our collective common sense ... we have so many wonderful new materials and techniques', and then went on to question whether 'we have the wisdom to use them appropriately'.[11]

The point being made was that the scientific rigour that was the basis of many preventive philosophies is 'not apparent in the current development of our restorative strategies'.

This view has been echoed by Brian Mouatt, the former Chief Dental Officer for England and Wales. He reflects on 'the frailty of human nature' in intervention, and states that 'some cures are not cures at all and may be totally ineffective, worse they may be harmful. Some techniques seem to work in the hands of some skilled operators, but when colleagues emulate their efforts, strangely, the reported results seem more elusive. Some techniques are applied more in hope than in certainty. Many are applied without the benefit of evidence to show that they are appropriate or useful.'[12]

Barriers to change

Research into the barriers to change has tended to focus on medical practice, and few studies have been conducted in dentistry. The following potential barriers to change have been identified:

- knowledge and attitudes of the practitioner
- patient factors

- practice environment
- educational environment
- wider health system
- social environment.

These factors apply equally to doctors and dentists.

We know that patients make value judgements when opting for a particular treatment in preference to another after discussing the options with their doctor or dentist.

The provision of endodontic treatment and periodontal treatment is influenced by patients' perspectives.[13]

The opinion of patients and fear of medico-legal actions are known to be influential factors in the dentist's decision to undertake bitewing radiography.[14]

Clearly, knowledge also plays an important part in the equation, and there is evidence to show that a range of procedures from the use of sealant restorations to endodontic treatment are directly influenced by the extent of a practitioner's commitment to continuing education.

One approach to overcoming these barriers recognises that:[15]

- behaviour change is a process
- change agents must identify with the clinician's concerns
- it is important to assess the stage of readiness for change and the specific nature of barriers to change
- multiple change strategies are more effective than single ones
- clinician education must include a focus on knowledge, attitudes and skill development
- educative strategies must be interactive and participatory
- social influence can be a powerful facilitator and inhibitor of behaviour change
- environmental support is crucial for the initiation and maintenance of change.

Some useful tips

The following tips[16] are the result of 17 projects across 15 health authorities. They provide a useful starting point for implementing changes based on research evidence in practice.

1 Select a topic where the evidence is conclusive and difficult to deny. It is essential to have total confidence in the evidence underpinning any changes you may wish to make.
2 Focus on changes that will have a visible effect and be widely welcomed by practice team members and patients.
3 Identify the best readily available indicators of impact or outcome, and measure these before, during and after the task. You may have to adopt a pragmatic approach to this, but it is important to have a yardstick to demonstrate the difference.
4 Look for and exploit natural links with other practitioners.

5   Tackle something realistic and achievable. Remember that sustainable change is most likely to be achieved when its implementation is incremental. Evolution is more effective than revolution.

Measuring clinical effectiveness

Measuring clinical effectiveness requires you to work systematically through the following stages:[17]

• asking the right question – framing it so that it is simple, specific, realistic, important, capable of being answered, owned by those involved, implementable, and focused on an area where change is possible
• finding the evidence – searching in the published literature, asking experts, etc.[18]
• weighing up the evidence – as applied to your question in relation to your situation
• applying the evidence in practice – involving others, linking practice and policies or strategic plans, getting ownership from work colleagues and managers, and overcoming barriers to application
• evaluating changes – making refinements to the application of evidence and continuing to monitor performance
• applying clinical effectiveness in the wider context of clinical governance.

Reviewing paper records may be slow and demanding, but it is a good place to start. Your existing records are a rich source of data.

Evidence-based patient education

Patients:

• want more information and seldom ask questions
• have difficulty remembering more than a few different messages at a time
• have different learning styles – some prefer written, spoken, audio information, etc.
• have different language, reading and comprehension abilities
• have a variety of life and health experiences.

Patient education materials have to reflect these observations, and should be sufficiently simple and flexible in the way that they are presented to fulfil a wide variety of needs for information and education.

Effective patient education programmes:

• reinforce desired outcomes and behaviours
• offer patients feedback on performance
• individualise materials to patients' wants, needs and preferences
• facilitate patients taking action for themselves
• are relevant to the patient's current problem

- allow patients to express negative thoughts and reactions to what is proposed
- help patients to feel in control.[19]

Patients' preferences and values must be considered alongside evidence-based care and dento-legal implications.

Information about the effectiveness of a treatment for patients might include the following:

- the likely effects of a particular intervention
- comparison of the risks and benefits of one intervention with others
- clear presentation of probabilities and uncertainties
- discussion of individual applicability
- appropriate inclusions and exclusions – justify range of interventions, options included
- discussion of professional and circumstantial biases
- cost.

Patients and the Internet

There is no doubt that patients use the World Wide Web to obtain information as a supplement or an alternative to consulting with healthcare professionals. Some of the reasons given for this include the following:

1   information-seeking behaviour to compensate for lack of information provided by their doctor or dentist
2   a lack of trust in their own doctor or dentist
3   an opportunity to ask questions anonymously
4   to compare and contrast the available treatment options
5   on advice from the practice, in cases where patients have expressed a particular interest in a particular field.

Better information improves patient care

Patients ought to be well enough informed to be in a position to make rational decisions about their treatment options. The better the information that patients receive, the better they are able to participate in making decisions about their own treatment and the alternatives. This focus on patient empowerment is a recurring theme within clinical governance. There is some evidence that well-informed patients who actively share in making decisions about their treatment have more favourable health outcomes.

Giving patients more information has been shown to be associated with greater patient satisfaction.[20] Patients were asked to evaluate 16 criteria of 'good practice'. Of these, eight were proposed by dentists and the other eight had been proposed by patients. 'Explanation of procedures' was ranked highest in the list proposed by patients.

Note

At the time of writing, the Editorial Board and publishers of *Evidence-Based Dentistry* are conducting a survey of dental practitioners to discover their opinions, needs and requests with regard to evidence-based dentistry and the journal.

Some ideas on who should do what to establish evidence-based practice and policy in your practice

The GDP

- Act as a good role model for the rest of the team with regard to adopting evidence-based practice and policy whenever possible.
- Consider whether new services and procedures will be clinically effective and cost-effective.
- Liaise with associates and hygienists to ensure that there is some degree of consistency in prescribing treatment options.
- Investigate information sources.

The dental hygienist

- Apply evidence-based clinical care in your everyday work, fitting in with the practice guidelines.
- Be sure of the evidence base for alternative approaches to providing care.

The practice manager

- Help to gather information about evidence-based practice.
- Organise this information in an easy-to-access format.
- Liaise with company representatives to gather material for clinicians to use and discuss in meetings.

The receptionist

- Help the practice team to monitor whether they are adopting evidence-based practice by gathering data under their direction.
- Keep up to date so that the information you give to patients about minor dental problems is based on evidence whenever possible.

References

1   Walker R and Certosimo F (2000) *Clinical Update.* **22**(1). Naval Postgraduate Dental School, MD.

2   NHS Executive (1996) *Promoting Clinical Effectiveness.* NHS Executive, Leeds.

3   Sackett DL, Rosenberg WM, Gray J *et al.* (1996) Evidence-based medicine: what it is, and what it isn't. *BMJ.* **312**: 71–2.

4   Mandel ID (1993) Clinical research – the silent partner in dental practice. *Quint Int.* **24**: 453–63.

5   Godlee F (1998) Getting evidence into practice (editorial). *BMJ.* **317**: 6.

6   Emling RC (1995) Understanding laboratory and clinical research: an overview. *J Clin Dent.* **6**: 157–60.

7   Editorial (1999) What type of filling? *Effective Healthcare.* **5**(2).

8   NHS Centre for Reviews and Dissemination (1999) *Getting Evidence into Practice. Effective Health Care Bulletin. Vol. 5.* Royal Society of Medicine Press, London.

9   Oxman AD, Thompson MA, Davis DA and Haynes RB (1995) No magic bullets: a systematic review of 102 trials of intervention to improve clinical practice. *Can Med Assoc J.* **153**: 1423–31.

10 McGlone P, Watt R and Sheiham A (2001) Evidence-based dentistry: an overview of the challenges in changing professional practice. *Br Dent J.* **190**(12): 636–9.

11 Robbins JW (1998) Evidence-based dentistry: what is it and what does it have to do with practice? *Quint Int.* **29**(12).

12 Mouatt B (1999) Looking for evidence. *The Dentist.* **June**.

13 Kay EJ and Blinkhorn AS (1996) A qualitative investigation of factors governing dentists' treatment philosophies. *Br Dent J.* **180**: 171–6.

14 Rushton VE, Horner K and Worthington HV (2002) Screening panoramic radiography of new adult patients: diagnostic yield when combined with bitewing radiography and identification of selection criteria. *Br Dent J.* **192**: 275–9.

15 Moulding NT, Silagy CA and Weller DP (1999) A framework for effective management of change in clinical practice: dissemination and implementation of clinical practice guide-lines. *Qual Health Care.* **8**: 177–83.

16 van Zwanenberg T and Harrison J (eds) (2000) *Clinical Governance in Primary Care.* Radcliffe Medical Press, Oxford.

17 Chambers R (1998) *Clinical Effectiveness Made Easy.* Radcliffe Medical Press, Oxford.

18 Carter Y and Falshaw M (eds) (1998) *Finding the Papers: a guide to Medline searching.* Radcliffe Medical Press, Oxford.

19 Nagle J and Streiffer R (1996) *Evidence-Based Patient Education. What really works?* Paper presented at Patient Education Conference, Nashville, TN.

20 Burke L and Croucher R (1996) Criteria of good dental practice generated by general dental practitioners and patients. *Int Dent J.* **46**: 3–9.

Action plan. Module 5: evidence-based practice and policy

Today's date: ....   Action plan to be completed by: ....

Tackled by	Identify need/assess problem	Plan of action: what will you do?/by when?
Individual – you		
Practice team – you and your colleagues		
Organisation – your practice		

Evaluation: evidence-based practice and policy

Complete an evaluation of progress by ....

Level of evaluation: perspective or work done on this component by	The need or problem	Outcome: what have you achieved?	Who was involved in doing it?	Evaluated: • by whom? • when? • what method was used?
Individual – you				
Practice team – you and your colleagues				
Organisation – your practice				

Record of your learning about 'evidence-based practice and policy'

Write in topic, date, time spent and type of learning activity

	Activity 1	Activity 2	Activity 3	Activity 4
In-house formal learning				
External courses				
Informal and personal				
Qualifications and/or experience gained				

MODULE 6

Confidentiality

The principle of confidentiality is basic to the practice of all healthcare. The Hippocratic Oath includes the declaration that 'all that may come to my knowledge in the exercise of my profession or outside of my profession which ought not to be spread abroad I will keep secret and will never reveal'.

The General Dental Council's view is:

> The dentist–patient relationship is founded on trust and a dentist should not disclose to a third party information about a patient acquired in a professional capacity without the permission of the patient.[1]

Patients attend for dental care in the belief that the information which they supply or which is found out about them during investigation or treatment will be kept secret.

The practice team has a responsibility to patients with whom they are in a professional relationship for the confidentiality and security of any information that is obtained. From experience, it is a widely held view that many aspects of confidentiality apply more to the medical profession than they do to the dental profession, and that strict adherence to the principles of confidentiality is somehow exaggerated in the latter.

However, 'if the [dental] profession expects to retain and place value on the disclosure by patients of such sensitive and necessary information as HIV status, or oral contraceptive use (in view of the possible suppressive effects of some antibiotics), its standards and probity should continue to be seen as equal to that of its sister professions.'[2]

The fundamental principle is that health professionals must not use or disclose any confidential information that is obtained in the course of their clinical work, other than for the clinical care of the patient to whom that information relates.

Exceptions to the above are as follows:

- if the patient consents to disclosure
- if it is in the patient's own interest that information should be disclosed, but it is either impossible or medically undesirable to seek their consent
- if the law requires (and does not merely permit) the health professional to disclose the information
- if the health professional has an overriding duty to society to disclose the information
- if the health professional agrees that disclosure is necessary in order to safeguard national security

- if the disclosure is necessary to prevent a serious risk to public health
- in certain circumstances, for the purposes of medical research.

Health professionals must be able to justify their decision to disclose information without consent. If you are in any doubt, consult with your professional indemnity organisation for advice.

Consent to disclosure

Information that is given to a health professional remains the property of the patient. Generally, consent is assumed for the *necessary* sharing of information with other professionals who are involved with the care of the patient for that episode of care or course of treatment and, where essential, for continuing care. Beyond this, informed consent must be obtained.

> A schoolteacher rings you about a particular pupil who is not at school because he says he has a dental appointment. The teacher asks your receptionist if this is true. Is your receptionist able to confirm or deny the fact that the pupil has an appointment?

Neither you nor your receptionist are in a position to disclose any information about the pupil if they are registered with you as a patient. You can contact the pupil (or their parents) and seek consent to do so, but not otherwise.

The development of modern information technology and the increasing amount of multidisciplinary teamwork in patient care make confidentiality difficult to uphold. You should be aware that patients often underestimate the amount of information sharing that occurs.

A paper reporting patients' expectations and attitudes showed considerable divergence from accepted practice.[3] The study was conducted in general medical practice, and it is accepted that patients may be far more sensitive about medical records than they would be about dental records, although the latter will contain the medical history of the patient. The results of this survey merit discussion on those grounds alone.

The majority of those interviewed felt that administrative and secretarial staff should not have access to their clinical records. Some of the patients had reservations about other doctors who were not directly concerned with their healthcare having access to their records. They were not aware of the extent to which other healthcare staff had access to their records.

Interestingly, Clause 68 of the Health and Social Care Bill gives the Secretary of State for Health powers to access medical records without a patient's consent, and they will also be able to pass on information to other organisations. Information from a patient's medical record may be shared with any organisation that the Secretary of State wishes, even if this is against the wishes of the patient or without their knowledge.

It is important to recognise that relatives or carers do *not* have any right to information about the patient. Do not breach confidentiality by giving information without consent (e.g. do not confirm a patient's attendance for treatment, or give any results of investigations to someone who states that they are a relative or carer).

Including information about confidentiality in the practice leaflet, and having notices about confidentiality displayed, help to inform patients about the standards that you set. Make sure that all of the staff understand the need for confidentiality, and explain to patients each time they ask for information the rules under which it is given.

Data Protection Act 1998

The main provisions of the Data Protection Act (1998) came into force on 1 March 2000. Although there are many similarities between this and the 1984 Act, some important differences should be recognised:

- the Act covers manual and electronic health records
- the Access to Health Records Act 1990 permitted access to manual records made after the Act came into force on 1 November 1991, but the Data Protection Act 1998 permits access to all manual records, whenever made (subject to specified exceptions)
- the eight data protection principles continue to apply but the nature of the principles differs between the two Acts. These are:
  1 'Personal data shall be processed fairly and lawfully and, in particular, shall not be processed unless at least one of the conditions in Schedule 2 is met, and in the case of sensitive personal data, at least one of the conditions in Schedule 3 is also met.'
  2 'Personal data shall be obtained only for one or more specified and lawful purposes, and shall not be further processed in any manner incompatible with that purpose or those purposes.'
  3 'Personal data shall be adequate, relevant and not excessive in relation to the purpose or purposes for which they are processed.'
  4 'Personal data shall be accurate and, where necessary, kept up to date.'
  5 'Personal data processed for any purpose or purposes shall not be kept for longer than is necessary for that purpose or those purposes.'
  6 'Personal data shall be processed in accordance with the rights of data subjects under this Act.'
  7 'Appropriate technical and organisational measures shall be taken against unauthorised or unlawful processing of personal data and against accidental loss or destruction of, or damage to, personal data.'
  8 'Personal data shall not be transferred to a country or territory outside the European Economic Area, unless that country or territory ensures an adequate level of protection for the rights and freedoms of data subjects in relation to the processing of personal data.'
- notification is now to the Data Protection Commissioner rather than the Data Protection Registrar as in the 1984 Act.

A health record for the purposes of the Act is one which relates to the physical or mental health of an individual which has been made by, or on behalf of, a health professional in connection with the care of that individual.

Teamwork issues

Increasingly, dentists are adopting a team approach to caring for their patients. Communication with other members of the team is essential. You may need to discuss explicitly with the patient what information will need to be made available to other members of the team. This will usually involve disclosure of a medical history that may be relevant to treatment provision.

Disclosure required by law

Confidential information may be required by law without the consent of the patient if an Act of Parliament says that it must be disclosed in some given circumstance or for some given purpose.

A Court Order may also order disclosure in a particular case. Failure to disclose information may then be illegal, although the health professional can still decline to do so on ethical grounds and risk the legal consequences (e.g. a fine or imprisonment).

If the legal requirements conflict with your ethical standpoint, seek advice from professional organisations and your professional indemnity provider.

Overriding duty to society

Occasionally you may feel that your moral duty as a citizen requires you to divulge confidential information. Whenever possible you should seek to persuade the patient to give consent to the disclosure. Seek advice from your professional organisations in circumstances where others are in danger (e.g. risk of harm, or rape or sexual abuse), or where a serious crime has been committed.

National security

Health professionals should satisfy themselves that sufficient authority has been obtained (e.g. a certificate from the Attorney General or Lord Advocate) and consult professional organisations before disclosing information without a patient's consent.

Public health

Legislation requires notification of certain diseases and conditions to the appropriate authorities. It may sometimes be necessary, in the public interest, to disclose information to prevent serious risks to other people's health (e.g. communicable diseases or adverse drug reactions).

You should satisfy yourself that information is passed to someone who has similar respect for confidentiality (not the media!).

Research

Increasingly, GDPs are being asked to participate in research in practice. For example, the Faculty of General Dental Practitioners (FGDP) encourages vocational dental practitioners to participate in research projects.

Research may benefit existing or future patients or lead to improvements in public health. Normally, confidential information about identified patients should not be used without their informed consent (*see* Module 3 on Establishing and disseminating a research and development culture).

The *Caldicott Committee Report*[4] describes the following principles of good practice to safeguard confidentiality when information is being used for non-clinical purposes.

- Justify the purpose.
- Do not use patient-identifiable information unless it is absolutely necessary to do so.
- Use the minimum necessary patient-identifiable information.
- Access to patient-identifiable information should be on a strict need-to-know basis.
- Everyone with access to patient-identifiable information should be aware of their responsibilities.

You should tell the patients whom you invite to participate in a consultation or survey about the standards of confidentiality. You should inform them about the extent to which their identity, contact details and the information that they give you is confidential to you, your work team or organisation.

If researchers approach you for data on patients from their records, you should not disclose it unless informed consent is given or that consent is not required after consideration by an appropriate ethical committee. You should not disclose information if you are aware that a patient would withhold their consent.

Teaching

The patient's informed consent should be obtained before any personal information required for the instruction is shared. Students should be made aware of the importance of confidentiality and its preservation. Intra-oral photography is frequently used for teaching and learning purposes, or as part of a case report prepared for submission for examination purposes, e.g. to the FGDP. Explain clearly to patients the purpose, use and audience, and give them an unpressurised opportunity to decline the use of this material if they are uncomfortable about it.

Confidentiality policy

A written confidentiality policy document should be drawn up and made known to all team members. Access to it should be encouraged, and supplementary guidance should be provided if there are any ambiguities.

A named person should be responsible for updating this policy document, monitoring adherence to it and dealing with any potential or actual breaches of confidentiality.

It should be noted that the policy extends to temporary, voluntary, dental or work-experience students, as well as equipment servicing engineers and technicians, all of whom should be informed of their obligations to maintain confidentiality.

In situations where friends, family or interpreters may be accompanying the patient, they should be aware of the confidentiality issues relating to the provision of treatment. If discussions are to take place with the patient, whether they are about clinical issues or financial matters relating to the cost of treatment, consent to discuss these in the presence of the third party should be sought first.

Security systems for paper and computer-held records should be regularly reviewed and upgraded.

Management, clerical and administrative staff responsibilities for confidentiality include the following:

- a clause about confidentiality in contracts of employment
- training in confidentiality for all staff
- a named person with whom any member of staff can discuss difficulties with confidentiality
- reporting physical difficulties, such as lack of privacy at reception desks or being overheard answering the telephone
- having clear rules about the handling of post marked 'private', 'confidential' or 'personal'
- explaining the reasons for requests for information from patients. Only seek the minimum amount of information required for the task
- shredding confidential paper records
- being particularly careful in situations where reception and waiting areas may be open plan.

Secure storage of records

The policy document on confidentiality should contain clear procedures for recording and storing information on paper or on computer. Safeguards against unauthorised access to either form of storage must be built in and tested.

Levels of access to data should be clearly stated, and passwords to computer records should be kept confidential (not left on a sticky label on the computer terminal). Terminal security must be arranged so that no unattended terminal can be used by an unauthorised person to access data.

Modem security must provide 'firewall' security against unauthorised access to confidential data. Technology makes sensitive data readily available – not just to those who need to access it.

Transmission of records and information

Consider the security of fax[5] or electronic data before using these methods of transmission. Do you know who will see the information at the other end?

When information is requested by telephone, do you know the identity of the person to whom you are speaking? Are you absolutely sure it is not a journalist pretending to be a patient? This has happened on a number of occasions when dentists have been involved in high-profile dento-legal cases.

Think about conflicts

- Medical information is confidential – yet employers and social security officers expect a signed diagnosis if someone is absent from work due to a dental problem.
- Medical information is confidential – yet a spouse may ask for details of the patient's treatment.
- Medical information is confidential – yet patients expect a full and informative letter to be sent with any request for a specialist opinion, although they may have reservations about secretaries or receptionists seeing their medical records.
- Medical information is confidential – yet patients give signed consent for their doctor to provide full details from their records to insurance companies, although they expect them to withhold harmful information.[6]

Some ideas on who should do what to establish confidentiality in your practice

The GDP

- Be clear about how to handle confidentiality, and adhere to recommended practice.
- Discuss patient details with other staff on a need-to-know basis.
- Do not talk about patients in public areas inside or outside the practice.
- Consult your defence organisation if you are unsure about releasing confidential information without the patient's authority if you are asked to do so.
- Include a clause on confidentiality in staff contracts of employment.

The practice manager

- Ensure that all staff are trained in the practice procedures for preserving confidentiality.
- Advertise how confidentiality is maintained in the practice leaflet and on posters.
- Monitor who has access to confidential records.
- Keep confidential staff records in a secure place.
- Review the practice procedures and the environment to anticipate how confidentiality might be breached.
- Help with training for members of the team.

The dental nurse

- Monitor others' access to patient records that are kept in treatment rooms.
- Monitor whether conversations or consultations in treatment rooms can be overheard.
- Do not talk about patients in areas where you can be overheard.

The receptionist

- Tell the practice manager if you think that patient requests can be overheard while you are on the telephone or at the desk.
- Always check identity and authorisation before releasing information.
- Report any worries or difficulties that you have with maintaining confidentiality.
- Take responsibility for shredding unwanted paper records of patient information.

References

1   General Dental Council (revised 2001) *Maintaining Standards. Para 3.5*. General Dental Council, London.

2   Matthews JBR (1995) *Risk Management in Dentistry*. Wright, Oxford.

3   Carman D and Britten N (1995) Confidentiality of medical records: the patient's perspective. *Br J Gen Pract.* **45**: 485–8.

4   Department of Health (1997) Report of the review of patient-identifiable information. In: *The Caldicott Committee Report*. Department of Health, London.

5   Genesen L *et al.* (1994) Faxing medical records: another threat to confidentiality in medicine. *JAMA.* **271**: 1401–2.

6   Lorge RE (1989) How informed is patient's consent to the release of medical information to insurance companies? *BMJ.* **298**: 1495–6.

Action plan. Module 6: confidentiality

Today's date: ....   Action plan to be completed by: ....

Tackled by	Identify need/assess problem	Plan of action: what will you do?/by when?
Individual – you		
Practice team – you and your colleagues		
Organisation – your practice		

Evaluation: confidentiality

Complete an evaluation of progress by ....

Level of evaluation: perspective or work done on this component by	The need or problem	Outcome: what have you achieved?	Who was involved in doing it?	Evaluated: • by whom? • when? • what method was used?
Individual – you				
Practice team – you and your colleagues				
Organisation – your practice				

Record of your learning about 'confidentiality'

Write in topic, date, time spent and type of learning activity

	Activity 1	Activity 2	Activity 3	Activity 4
In-house formal learning				
External courses				
Informal and personal				
Qualifications and/or experience gained				

MODULE 7

Health gain

Definitions

It has been said that 'health is one of a number of words that are constantly in use which are so rich in meaning that they cannot be explained fully without involving controversy'. To try to define health is to enter a philosophical and scientific quagmire. What might have been accepted as health a few years ago may today be an unacceptable definition. Then there are the intangible elements, such as expectations, aesthetics and conflicting scientific discovery, all of which combine to add to the 'spin' about health but may not address the core issues of 'substance'. The pre-eminent French historian and philosopher Georges Canguilhem noted that health was 'essentially a negative state rather than a positive one; when one is healthy one is oblivious of the issue of health or ill health as a problem'. The World Health Organization defines it as 'a state of complete physical, mental and social well-being, not merely the absence of disease or handicap'.

There are two general approaches to improving health:

1   the 'population approach' – focusing on measures to improve health throughout the community
2   the 'high-risk' approach – concentrating on those at highest risk of ill health.

This approach is reflected in the structure and development of dental services, where the General Dental Service (GDS) and Community Dental Service (CDS) have broadly reflected these approaches.

The two approaches are not mutually exclusive, and often need to be combined with legislation and community action.

The Nation's Health: a strategy for the 1990s[1] sets out priority areas and detailed action plans for each of them. The authors list eight important general principles for public health strategies:

1   partnership between public, professionals and policy makers
2   co-ordination between different organisations
3   adequate funding
4   long-term planning
5   recognising barriers to health promotion

6   reducing inequalities in health
7   education for health
8   research, evaluation and monitoring.

The health gain strategy has three interdependent parts, all of which are covered in this module.

Resources for health

We must accept that resources are limited and dentists should have some input and understanding of how resources are allocated at both local and national levels. Effective use of resources is an important part of clinical governance, but we do it every day in general practice. We have to manage the business and deliver a high standard of care within our pre-determined range of resources.

The management of these resources produces two outcomes. First, there will be patient groups for whom the practice will provide a comprehensive service and whose needs will be looked after. Secondly, there may also be patients who as a result of decisions about how resources are allocated may be excluded for reasons of cost or any other potentially divisive practice policy.

Evaluation and feedback

Policy strategy has to provide channels for evaluation and feedback. Good-quality data collection is essential for adequate evaluation (*see* Module 4 on Reliable and accurate data).

Audit and research

Audit enables you to monitor whether you are doing what you set out to do.

Adequate funding

An adequate income for everyone is beyond the control and influence of health workers, but would have a major impact on public health. From the perspective of clinical practice, we are only too aware that inequalities of health are closely related to poverty, poor housing and poor education.[2,3] Funding for resources and services is always inadequate compared with what could be done. Attempts to prop up the NHS (e.g. the Modernisation Fund) have helped, but there is the view that it is too little, too late.

Innovations for quality improvements

The 1997 White Paper *The New NHS: modern, dependable*[4] promised to put quality at the heart of the health service. It introduced the following:

- the National Institute for Clinical Excellence (NICE) to promote work on clinical and cost-effectiveness at national level and to draw up and disseminate guidelines. The guidance on removal of third molars is an early example
- the Commission for Health Improvement (CHI) to support and oversee the quality of services at local level
- National Service Frameworks (NSFs) – evidence-based guidance to help to ensure consistent access to services and quality of care
- clinical governance in NHS trusts and throughout the rest of the NHS, backed by statutory provisions and designed to 'put quality on the agenda' of every NHS trust board
- a survey of patients' experiences of NHS care as an annual review.

The consultative document *A First-Class Service: quality in the new NHS*[5] gives a more detailed description of the planned changes. GDPs have greeted the pronouncements with caution. The widely held view is that the changes imposed on the NHS by the Government have tended to be reactive to scandal or outrage rather than proactive in the systematic pursuit of excellence.

Improving Health Care[6] outlines several difficulties with the proposed policy.

- The NICE agenda needs to include the development of evidence-based approaches to health risk reduction, early disease screening and other public health improvements. Evidence other than that generated by randomised controlled trials may need to be considered to prevent bias in the development of service provision.
- Little information exists on NHS users' qualitative care experiences. The annual survey of patients' experiences may provide new information, but other specific enquiries may need to be made.
- Evaluation techniques are unreliable, and new ways of assessing performance need to be developed. Effective self-help instruments for improving the performance of health-care organisations, units and professionals should be developed.
- The expectations of better services conflict with tight financial controls.
- Over-regulation undermines the ability of health professionals to do their jobs properly.
- Quality management is not free.
- Obtaining opinions from patients' representatives is not the same as giving individuals opportunities to participate fully in improving their personal health. Better self-care is the basis for almost all good healthcare.

GDPs can identify with all of these concerns from their experience of running their own practices.

Changing behaviour

What about telling people to change their behaviour? It sounds straightforward, but is there any evidence that it works?

For example, a study from the USA[7] indicated that drug prevention programmes targeted towards teenagers could produce meaningful and long-lasting reductions in tobacco, alcohol and marijuana use. Using data from the whole sample of 3597 students, the effects of both intervention programmes were to reduce cigarette consumption significantly – a reduction of 6% (from 33% to 27%) using cigarettes in any month. The proportion smoking 20 cigarettes a day was reduced by more than 20%. There was no difference in overall alcohol use, although problem drinking was reduced significantly (by 6%). There were only slight differences in marijuana consumption.

Viewed by the overall results alone, the gains of preventive interventions may seem small. However, these results were obtained *six years after the intervention*, and they show powerful and long-lasting effects of an intensive and thorough prevention programme incorporating social skills training. Even modest gains spread over a large population can have immense health gains for society and individuals.

It was notable that the programmes had a much greater impact in the subgroup that attended more than 60% of the classes. Heavy smoking, heavy drinking and polydrug use were reduced substantially (by 25% to 66%). These are large and significant health gains.

This study was randomised, intensive and had a long period of follow-up. All of those involved in the design and implementation of health prevention programmes should read up on this study.

We know that there have been numerous attempts at and initiatives for changing behaviour, and some of them have been more successful than others.

Do you still believe that people do not change their behaviour as a result of your efforts? Have a look at the Cochrane Review on the effectiveness of advice for smoking cessation.[8]

Individual efforts to give advice on smoking cessation targeted at health service users need to be coupled with population-directed health promotion activities. These include Government measures such as taxation, control of sales, health warnings, control of advertising, funding for health promotion and smoking cessation programmes that involve healthcare providers. Media coverage should include free comment on the dangers of smoking without undue pressure from advertisers, and fictional characters should reflect the increased majority of non-smokers in the population. Local policies on non-smoking at work have proved to be highly successful and could be extended to more social meeting places.

Whether we are talking about oral health and hygiene or the wider issues of general health, the principles remain the same.

However, there are other issues that also need to be addressed. Consider a GDP who decides to impose sanctions on treatments. In other words, treatment will be available only if there are certain behavioural changes in place first. Examples might include construction of a bridge for a patient whose oral hygiene is unsatisfactory, or the provision of implants for a patient who continues to smoke heavily. The challenge is to identify who decides on what constitutes ethical provision of care and treatment. Does the practitioner have ownership of the patient's health? If the answer is clearly no, then how does that relate to the ethical issue of duty of care?

The social and cultural norms have to be recognised.[9] 'The application of sanctions against a patient, or making an individual feel guilty about their inability to put into practice what is recommended, could cause harm to them and offend against the ethical principle of non-maleficence.'

Looking for the evidence of health gain

What is it that we are trying to measure? The definition of oral health proposed by the Department of Health[10] gives us some direction, but it can be interpreted in many ways: 'Oral health is the standard of health of the oral and related tissues which enables an individual to eat, speak and socialise without active disease, discomfort or embarrassment, and which contributes to general well-being.'

Interestingly, the definition is patient centred and is now widely accepted internationally. One way of looking for that evidence of gain is to consider what is important to you and your patient, and you may want to consider an encounter with a patient as a good place to start (*see* Figure M7.1).

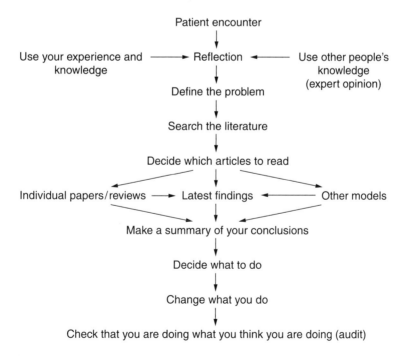

Figure M7.1   Looking for evidence of health gain.

Good places to look for information on evidence of health gain include the following:

- *Bandolier* (www.jr2.ox.ac.uk/bandolier/subind.html)
- The York Centre for Effective Health Care (www.york.ac.uk/inst.crd)
- The ScHaRR site, which lists many others (www.shef.ac.uk/~scharr/ir/netting.html)

Measuring health gain

The different types of evidence available can be ranked according to how authoritative they are (*see* Module 5 on Evidence-based practice and policy). In a similar way, the effectiveness of an intervention may be judged in terms of its potential to deliver health gain. The health gain ranking is as follows:

1   *beneficial* – where the effectiveness can be clearly demonstrated
2   *likely to be beneficial* – where the effectiveness is not so firmly established
3   *trade-off between beneficial and adverse effects* – where the effects are weighed up according to individual circumstances
4   *unknown* – where there is insufficient information to recommend the intervention
5   *unlikely to be beneficial* – where the ineffectiveness is not as clearly demonstrated as for (6) below
6   *likely to be ineffective or harmful* – where ineffectiveness or potential for harm is clearly demonstrated.

For example, in the *Health Evidence Bulletin*[11] the statement is made that 'sugar substitutes may be of benefit in reducing dental caries. However, other effects of such substitutes should be understood and taken into account.' This statement carries an 'unknown' rating on this scale because the evidence to support the view is from intervention studies without randomisation. The ranking suggests the need for more robust evidence.

The Oral Health Index

The Oral Health Index (OHX) was developed in the early 1990s[12] and was based on the Oral Health Strategy Group's definition quoted earlier. This concept was developed to create an Oral Health Index that is now widely used as part of the Denplan Excel programme.[13]

The oral health score has been modified to simplify the calculation of the final index, which now includes eight components. There is a protocol in place within the Denplan Excel programme in line with the original work on the index. This is summarised in Table M7.1 opposite.

The maximum possible score is 100. The index is patient centred, and if there is any doubt about how to score the categories of pain, appearance and chewing ability, the patient should be asked to score the importance of the problem him- or herself.

Table M7.1   The Oral Health Score (reproduced by kind permission of Mike Busby and Denplan)

Component	What to do	Basis of scoring
Pain	Ask the patient if they have any pain	No pain = 8 Minor problems = 4 Disruptive pain = 0
Chewing ability	Ask the patient to what extent they can chew an unrestricted diet	Yes = 8 Minor problems = 4 Major disruption = 0
Appearance	Ask the patient if anything concerns them about the appearance of their teeth	No problems = 8 Minor problems = 4 Major problems = 0
Oral mucosa	Examine the mucosa	No lesions detected = 8 Lesions requiring observation only = 4 Lesions requiring active treatment = 0
Occlusion	Examine the dentition	A minimum of 10 teeth (artificial or natural) are present in each jaw and they oppose each other = 8 Otherwise = 0
Caries	Examine the mouth in sextants	Score each sextant free from active caries requiring restoration as 4 Score any sextant containing a tooth with active caries requiring restoration as 0
Periodontal disease	Examine the periodontal tissues	Start with a score of 24. From this maximum score delete the BPE score for each sextant

The score is also a useful communication tool, and in addition it provides information and could be used as a measure of health gain or as a performance indicator.

Preventive services for oral health

Screening procedures are used to try to detect illness before it develops. Wilson's criteria[14] help us to decide whether screening is worthwhile. A useful mnemonic from Clarke and Croft[15] is shown in the box overleaf.

   Screening for oral cancer provides one example. In the case of oral cancer, detection may fail for any of the following reasons:

*   There is no systematic way of carrying out the check in the practice.
*   Patients do not attend.

Wilson's criteria for screening: TRAP WILSON

Treatable condition
Resources for screening and treatment available
Activity must be continuous
Audit cycle continued
Protocols needed for a clear policy on when to treat
Worthwhile (cost versus benefit)
Important to individual and community
Latent phase exists for detection before disease develops
Suitable and acceptable test
Outcome improved by detection
Natural history well understood

- The condition developed after the last consultation.
- The test did not detect the cancer (a false-negative result was obtained either because of failure to take the sample from the area of the cancer, or because the test result was read incorrectly).

Working practices

You may be prompted to review your approach by a challenge from a patient or colleague about the usefulness of what you are promoting.

For example, you may be recommending that the patient has simple periodontal therapy with your hygienist at, say, three-monthly intervals, and the patient questions the value of this service. You may need to look up the current guidelines on maintaining gingival health and review your practice and procedures accordingly and, equally importantly, be able to communicate the findings to your patient. This may mean producing an information leaflet to help them to understand your perspective.

Other reasons why you may need to review your working practices could include the following:

- a critical incident
- a complaint
- adverse criticism from a colleague, patient or authority figure
- an audit that shows poor compliance with national or local guidelines
- the introduction of new techniques and/or materials.

See Module 5 on Evidence-based practice and policy, Module 8 on Coherent teamwork and Module 10 on Meaningful patient involvement.

Some ideas on who should do what to achieve health gain in your practice

The GDP

- Incorporate national priorities into practice working.
- Learn new ways of influencing behaviour.
- Focus on improving access for high-risk and disease-susceptible patients.
- Ensure that the nurses to whom you may delegate dental health education initiatives are adequately trained to accept the tasks and responsibilities and have the resources to undertake them.

The practice manager

- Identify the changes needed when new procedures are introduced.
- Identify staff training needs when change occurs.

The hygienist

- Develop more sophisticated approaches to dental health education.
- Keep good records so that you can remind at-risk groups about follow-up if they default.
- Develop protocols for devolved care.

The receptionist

- Be flexible when high-risk patients ask for an appointment or prescription.
- Monitor the attendance of high-risk patients and follow up patients who fail to attend.

References

1   Jacobson B, Smith A and Whitehead M (1991) *The Nation's Health: a strategy for the 1990s.* King Edward's Hospital Fund for London, London.

2   Black D (1980) *Inequalities in Health. Report of a research working group.* Department of Health and Social Security, London.

3   Whitehead M (1988) The health divide. In: *Inequalities in Health.* Penguin, Harmondsworth.

4   Department of Health (1997) *The New NHS: modern, dependable.* The Stationery Office, London.

5   Department of Health (1998) *A First-Class Service: quality in the new NHS*. Department of Health, London.

6   Taylor D (1998) *Improving Health Care*. King's Fund Publishing, London.

7   Botvin GJ, Baker E, Dusenbury L, Botvin EM and Diaz T (1995) Long-term follow-up of a randomized drug abuse prevention trial in a white middle-class population. *JAMA*. **273**: 1106–12.

8   Lancaster T, Silagy C, Fowler G and Spiers I (1999) Training health professionals in smoking cessation. In: *The Cochrane Library*. Update Software, Oxford.

9   Gibbons DE (2002) Resource allocation and business ethics. In: P Lambden (ed.) *Dental Law and Ethics*. Radcliffe Medical Press, Oxford.

10   Department of Health (1994) *Oral Health Strategy*. Department of Health, London.

11   Welsh Office (1988) *Wales Oral Health Protocol Enhancements Project*. Welsh Office of Research and Development for Health and Social Care, Welsh Office, Cardiff.

12   Burke FTJ and Wilson NHF (1995) Measuring oral health: an historical view and details of a contemporary oral health index. *Int Dent J*. **45**: 358–70.

13   Denplan Excel Accreditation Programme. Denplan, Winchester.

14   Wilson JMG (1976) Some principles of early diagnosis and detection. In: G Teeling-Smith (ed.) *Proceedings of a Colloquium, Magdalen College, Oxford*. Office of Health Economics, London.

15   Clarke R and Croft P (1998) *Critical Reading for the Reflective Practitioner*. Butterworth-Heinemann, Oxford.

Action plan. Module 7: health gain

Today's date: ....   Action plan to be completed by: ....

Tackled by	Identify need/assess problem	Plan of action: what will you do?/by when?
Individual – you		
Practice team – you and your colleagues		
Organisation – your practice		

Evaluation: health gain

Complete an evaluation of progress by ....

Level of evaluation: perspective or work done on this component by	The need or problem	Outcome: what have you achieved?	Who was involved in doing it?	Evaluated: • by whom? • when? • what method was used?
Individual – you				
Practice team – you and your colleagues				
Organisation – your practice				

Record of your learning about 'health gain'

Write in topic, date, time spent and type of learning activity

	Activity 1	Activity 2	Activity 3	Activity 4
In-house formal learning				
External courses				
Informal and personal				
Qualifications and/or experience gained				

Coherent teamwork

The importance of good teamwork has been emphasised in many recent Government documents.[1-3] Teams do produce better patient care than single practitioners operating in a fragmented way.[4]

Effective teams make the most of the different contributions of individual clinical disciplines in delivering patient care. The characteristics of effective teams are as follows:

- shared ownership of a common purpose
- clear goals for the contributions that each discipline makes
- open communication between team members
- opportunities for team members to enhance their skills.

A team approach helps different team members to adopt an evidence-based approach to patient care – by having to justify their approach to the rest of the team.[4]

Teamwork and the vision for primary care

The themes[5] that are emerging as a future vision of healthcare delivery are centred on teams with:

- boundaries between primary and secondary care disappearing
- more integrated care
- more user-friendly primary care (as is being developed through *NHS Direct* and Dental Access centres)
- easier access to primary care
- an increased range of healthcare services provided by primary care practitioners in primary care settings
- an increasingly multidisciplinary primary care workforce
- nurses with extended skills, responsibilities and training
- continuing gatekeeping responsibilities in primary care
- greater integration between health and social services planning and provision.

The scope for teamwork in general dental practice has been severely restricted by legislation, but at its meeting in November 2001, the General Dental Council (GDC) approved proposals for a new statutory framework for the dental team as a whole. Developed in close consultation with a number of dental associations/organisations, at the time of writing the proposals are under consideration by the Department of Health.

At present the regulatory remit of the GDC extends to dentists, dental hygienists and dental therapists, but there are plans to expand this to include the following:

- dental nurses
- dental technicians/clinical dental technicians
- maxillofacial prosthetists and technologists
- orthodontic therapists.

This means that all professionals complementary to dentistry (PCDs) will be recognised as professionals, and the proposals appear to have received the approval of the Government. Consequently, there will be:

- approved training courses for all members of the dental team
- a range of public protection measures
- ethical guidance for all team members – based on responsibilities for which they have received appropriate training
- established standards for inclusion on a register – there is likely to be a single PCD register.

The aim is to roll out registration of dental team members new to statutory registration in 2003–04 with a framework which is built on curricula and ethical guidance, rather than on restricted lists of duties. This would be a ground-breaking event destined to reshape the delivery of dental services in primary care.

Teamwork will be necessary to deliver clinical governance

Teamwork is central to the success of any general dental practice. From a clinical governance perspective, teams can be involved in the following:

1 *protecting patients* by:
   - registration of PCDs
   - risk management.
2 *developing people* by:
   - continuing professional development
   - increasing their awareness of current 'best practice' guidelines
   - recognising and rewarding success.
3 *developing teams and systems* by:
   - learning from what other teams do well
   - clinical audit

- a commitment to evidence-based clinical practice
- improving cost-effectiveness
- listening to the views of patients
- participating in practice accreditation programmes.

Many of these concepts and aspirations are not new, but putting them together as a whole is a new approach for the NHS.

Effective teams

Team effectiveness relates to:

- teamworking methods
- practice efficiency
- individual motivation
- patient-centred care.

However, this is only one way of looking at what different bodies mean by 'effectiveness'[6] in relation to teamwork, because different organisations have different perspectives on the meaning of 'effectiveness', as shown in the table below.

Constituency	Examples of criteria for rating team effectiveness
Patients	Quality of service
Staff	Work satisfaction, pay, skill and career development
Hospitals	Appropriate referrals, communication
Strategic health authorities	Target achievement, data collection, efficient use of resources
Department of Health	Target achievement, consumer satisfaction, efficient use of resources
Professional organisations	Quality of service, skill level/skill mix of staff, career development of individual members

Teams that encourage participation, are more likely to achieve a patient-centred service, to work together as a team and be more efficient.[1]

All of the team members should determine the objectives for the team.

Your team is more likely to function well if it:[2]

- has clear team goals and objectives
- has clear lines of accountability and authority
- has diverse skills and personalities
- has specific individual roles for members
- shares tasks
- regularly communicates within the team, both formally and informally
- has full participation by team members
- confronts conflict

- monitors team objectives
- gives feedback to individuals
- gives feedback on team performance
- has external recognition of the team
- has two-way external communication between the team and the outside world
- offers rewards for the team.

A team leader with a democratic style enables a team to function well[7] and encourages rather than imposes change.

Good communication in teams

Good communication is essential for good teamwork.[8] You need:

- regular staff meetings – which managers and staff endeavour to attend
- a failsafe system for passing on important messages
- a way to share news so that everyone is promptly notified of changes
- a culture where team members can speak openly without fear of being judged or reprimanded
- opportunities for quieter members of the team to contribute
- to give and receive feedback on how your role in the team is working out
- to praise others for their achievements
- opportunities for team members to point out problems and suggest improvements
- everyone to be part of, and to own, the decision making.

Communication is usually poor if a team lacks stability, and power and status issues within a team can interfere with good communication.

Innovations are more likely in teams that communicate well. Innovative teams:[9]

- collaborate
- have committed teamworkers
- tolerate diversity
- communicate well
- have practical support
- give encouragement.

Integrated teams

A detailed study of integrated nursing teams produced the following findings.[10]

Good points

- The team was highly structured, problem focused and goal orientated.
- Multiprofessional practices such as note keeping, assessment, monitoring and evaluation were common.
- Team members were willing to be flexible about their roles.
- Being a team player was as important as being a member of a particular discipline.
- A learning culture was facilitated and supported by the heads of departments.

Not so good points

- Not all team members were clear and confident about their roles.
- Problem-solving skills varied within the team.
- Although teaching between professionals was common, nurses seemed to be excluded from a teaching role.
- It was difficult to integrate a newcomer into the team because she had a different philosophy about teamworking.

Integrated teams may not be exclusive to nurses. One multidisciplinary integrated team attributed their success to the professional:[2]

- being prepared to demonstrate their skills so that all team members could observe what each was doing
- being clear about their role and contribution
- being flexible about working across role boundaries where necessary.

The benefits of this integrated teamworking were as follows:

- *for patients* – continuity, consistency, appropriate referrals, less ambiguity, holistic information, better problem solving
- *for team members* – professional development through exchange of knowledge and skills.

The organisational factors that facilitate integrated teamwork can be summarised as follows:[10]

- working close together
- having a stable environment
- being able to predict what happens
- being a specialist team
- having supportive management structures
- having matching organisational policies.

Your practice may not have all of these ingredients in your team; in these studies, cohesion was the essential ingredient for successful integrated teamwork, so work on that first in your own work situation (*see* Module 1 on Establishing and sustaining a learning culture).

Teambuilding

When power is well managed, it can encourage security, support and trust with frank and open discussion and negotiation – all part of *teambuilding*.[8]

Teambuilding starts from the top. GDPs and practice managers should set good examples that encourage trust and respect from other colleagues. Without this, no practice is able to function at its full potential. This takes time, effort and consistency, but you will reap the rewards.

Teams may break down as a result of poor management, lack of guidance, poor communication and poor support.

Experienced practitioners will be only too aware of the games and ploys that are instigated by people who want to hang on to power, who may feel insecure or threatened by others. Remember that power is a *bargaining chip* that people will try to grab, steal or manipulate. When power in any practice is abused or mismanaged, the results will inevitably lead to a dysfunctional work environment. This can lead to the same troubles as beset a dysfunctional family – it falls apart. The consequences of this can be devastating to the efficient running of a dental practice, and will undoubtedly affect the quality of care that is provided for patients.

Unless the difficulties are acknowledged, and the practice is fully committed to the concept of teambuilding, attempts to improve the situation are likely to be a waste of time and resources.

Skill mix

Skill mix is not an arrangement where a less skilled colleague is substituted for another, or where one discipline is substituted for another, such as a hygienist taking a dentist's place.

'Multiskilling', where several professionals develop their roles in generic ways, is not the same as multiprofessional working, where team members meet to discuss and understand each other's roles and responsibilities, learn together and plan team strategies. Recent examples of skill substitution include the telephone helpline service, *NHS Direct*, and the primary care Walk-in centres, all staffed by nurses who provide the first point of contact in helping and advising patients.

The integrated primary care team of the future[11] might have fewer health professionals but with a more appropriate skill mix providing care. An appropriately skilled team will co-ordinate the different health, social and voluntary disciplines. It may have input from financial advisers, housing and transport officers and other relevant services. There could be several skilled subteams within the overarching primary care team.

Some of these issues are explored in *Options for Change*, due for publication in late 2002.

The team function test

Good teamwork does not just happen. Take time out as a team away from the workplace to review how you are working together. Everyone should have an equal opportunity to give their perspective on how the team is functioning.

Take the challenge below:[8]

There is good communication between colleagues at work	*usually*	*seldom*	*not at all*
There is good communication between managers and staff	*usually*	*seldom*	*not at all*
Team members' functions are clear	*usually*	*seldom*	*not at all*
Staff are proud to be working in your practice/unit	*usually*	*seldom*	*not at all*
Dentists/managers resolve staff problems	*usually*	*seldom*	*not at all*
Staff are treated with respect by the dentists	*usually*	*seldom*	*not at all*
There is a person-friendly culture at work	*usually*	*seldom*	*not at all*
There are opportunities for self-improvement for staff	*usually*	*seldom*	*not at all*
Positive feedback about performance is the norm at work	*usually*	*seldom*	*not at all*
Staff are well trained for the tasks they are asked to do	*usually*	*seldom*	*not at all*
Team members' responsibilities are clear	*usually*	*seldom*	*not at all*
There is good leadership in your team	*usually*	*seldom*	*not at all*

Score: usually = 3, seldom = 1, not at all = 0.
Scores between 27 and 36: you have a well-functioning team.
Scores between 24 and 15: *look at your weak areas and make plans for improvements.*
Scores between 15 and 0: *as you have a long way to go, it may be best for you to consider using an external consultant to help to facilitate team development.*

Some ideas on who should do what to establish a coherent practice team

The GDP

- Be a more democratic leader.
- Encourage multiprofessional working; value individual members' contributions to the team.
- Keep to the objectives set by the team; don't go your own way when it suits you.
- Join in multiprofessional learning and training with other team members.

The practice manager

- Make sure that you not only understand the characteristics of effective teams, but also positively create those factors in your team.

- Involve all team members and keep in regular communication with them.
- Put teamwork at the heart of clinical governance.
- Arrange regular staff meetings and encourage everyone to participate.
- Give feedback and praise to team members when it is due – remember to praise in public but criticise in private.

The dental nurse

- Be flexible about fitting in with new requirements for different ways of working.
- Collaborate with other team members to find more efficient ways of working.
- Don't allow your status to get in the way of teamworking.

The receptionist

- Try to attend staff meetings.
- Contribute your views and suggestions – your ideas are just as valuable as everyone else's.
- Don't forget to pass on messages and news to other team members.

The hygienist

- Blend in with the team and fit in with their objectives and strategy.
- Contribute to staff meetings.
- Agree your role and responsibilities in looking after patients with chronic periodontal diseases with others in the team.

References

1　NHS Executive (1997) *The New NHS: modern, dependable*. NHS Executive, Leeds.

2　NHS Executive (1998) *Working Together: securing a quality workforce for the NHS*. NHS Executive, Leeds.

3　NHS Executive (1999) *Patient and Public Involvement in the New NHS*. NHS Executive, Leeds.

4　Dunning M, Abi-Aad G, Gilbert D *et al.* (1999) *Experience, Evidence and Everyday Practice*. King's Fund, London.

5　Coffey T, Boersma G, Smith I and Wallace P (eds) (1999) *Visions of Primary Care*. King's Fund, London.

6　Poulton B and West M (1999) The determinants of effectiveness in primary health care teams. *J Interprof Care*. **13**: 7–18.

7   Hart E and Fletcher J (1999) Learning how to change: a selective analysis of literature and experience of how teams learn and organisations change. *J Interprof Care.* **13**: 53–63.

8   Chambers R and Davies M (1999) *What Stress in Primary Care!* Royal College of General Practitioners, London.

9   West M and Wallace M (1991) Innovation in health care teams. *Eur J Soc Psychol.* **21**: 303–15.

10 Miller C, Ross N and Freeman M (1999) *Shared Learning and Clinical Teamwork: new directions in education and multiprofessional practice.* English National Board for Nursing, Midwifery and Health Visiting, University of Brighton, Brighton.

11 NHS Alliance (2000) *Implementing the Vision.* NHS Alliance, Nottingham.

Action plan. Module 8: coherent teamwork

Today's date: ....   Action plan to be completed by: ....

Tackled by	Identify need/assess problem	Plan of action: what will you do?/by when?
Individual – you		
Practice team – you and your colleagues		
Organisation – your practice		

Evaluation: coherent teamwork

Complete an evaluation of progress by ....

Level of evaluation: perspective or work done on this component by	The need or problem	Outcome: what have you achieved?	Who was involved in doing it?	Evaluated: • by whom? • when? • what method was used?
Individual – you				
Practice team – you and your colleagues				
Organisation – your practice				

Record of your learning about 'coherent teamwork'

Write in topic, date, time spent and type of learning activity

	Activity 1	Activity 2	Activity 3	Activity 4
In-house formal learning				
External courses				
Informal and personal				
Qualifications and/or experience gained				

MODULE 9

Audit and evaluation

Audit has been described as 'the method used by health professionals to assess, evaluate and improve the care of patients in a systematic way, to enhance their health and quality of life'.[1] The five steps of the audit cycle are as follows:

1 Describe the criteria and standards that you are trying to achieve.
2 Measure your current performance with regard to how well you are providing care or services in an objective way.
3 Compare your performance against the criteria and standards.
4 Identify the need for change – to performance, adjustment of criteria or standards, resources, available data.
5 Make any required changes as necessary, and re-audit later.

The report *Modernising NHS Dentistry: clinical audit and peer review in the GDS* described clinical audit (and peer review) as a 'central pillar of clinical governance' and outlined the requirement to undertake a total of 15 hours in each successive period of three years. Dentists working in the General Dental Service (GDS) (irrespective of their level of commitment) are entitled to claim loss of earnings for a maximum of 15 hours over this three-year period. Participation in this scheme can also count towards the GDC's verifiable CPD requirement.

Performance is often broken down into the three aspects of structure, process and outcome for the purposes of audit.[2]

Structural audits might concern resources such as equipment, premises, skills, people, etc. *Process* audits focus on what was done to the patient, such as clinical protocols and guidelines. Audits of *outcomes* consider the impact of care or services on the patient, and might include patient satisfaction, health gains, and effectiveness of treatment or services. This presents a major challenge to the dental profession, because 'outcomes are conceptualised in different ways ... disease, disability, discomfort and dissatisfaction'.[1]

There are also many factors that combine to deliver clinical outcomes, including the general health of the patient, motivation, the skills of the clinician, effective communication, demographic factors, lifestyle factors and patient susceptibility to disease. Any combination of these may combine to give a particular outcome in one patient, but a different outcome in another patient. This is the challenge of *attribution,* and it is the experience of many GDPs that dental health outcomes are influenced by factors that are beyond the control of the clinician.

Furthermore, there may not necessarily be a direct relationship between structure, process and outcome, but the assumption is made that it would be difficult to deliver high-quality care in a failing environment where, for example, staffing levels may be inadequate and the equipment is out of date or unreliable. *See* Module 3 on Establishing and disseminating a research and development culture.

Purpose of audit

The purpose of an internal clinical audit is to fulfil a range of functions, including the following:

*   monitoring compliance with statutory requirements
*   monitoring adherence to clinical guidelines
*   monitoring adherence to non-clinical but necessary operational processes and systems in the practice
*   minimising and managing clinical and non-clinical risk
*   identifying learning needs by revealing gaps in skills and knowledge
*   minimising stress at work
*   maintaining the viability of the practice.

Any number or combination of functions can be fulfilled depending on what topic is selected for audit.

An audit protocol (*see* Chapter 3)

Follow this protocol to help you carry out the audit on an important topic.

1   Choose a topic that is a priority for you. What is it?

2   What problem are you addressing?

3   How did you choose the topic?

    *   *in discussion with other colleagues*
    *   *decided on behalf of my work colleagues*
    *   *the practice team requested the topic*
    *   *topic is in the business or strategic plan.*

4   Why did you choose this topic? Is it a priority topic? *Yes/No*
    If *yes*, is it a priority for (circle all that apply) the district's Health Improvement and Modernisation Plan (HIMP), the Government, the locality, the trust, the health authority, the primary care trust, patients, the community, workplace colleagues, self, the profession, National Service Framework (NSF), National Institute for Clinical

Excellence (NICE), previous/recent significant event (organisational, clinical or performance), other (please write in):

5   Is the topic important? (circle all that apply): *Yes/No*
    If *yes*, is it high cost, a common problem, a population need, a routine check of everyday care or services? Is there evidence that current standards are inadequate?
    Are there any other reasons why it is important to audit this topic?

6   What changes do you hope to make? Please write them here:

7   Are these changes possible with your current resources and skills? Are you being realistic in expecting change? From where will you obtain any additional resources?

8   What will you do? Try to make sure that you include as many of the principles of good practice in clinical governance as possible, which are to:

    •   have input from colleagues as appropriate
    •   consider the patient's perspective
    •   be capable of achieving health gains
    •   be based on evidence-based practice, policy or management principles.

Audit action plan

You can use the following to help you develop your audit action plan.

•   Who will lead the audit initiative?

•   Who else will be involved?

•   What resources do you need to undertake the audit?

•   What criteria have you selected and why?

•   What standards have you selected and from where did they originate?
    You may want to ask yourself some searching questions in this respect.
    Are they 'arbitrary' standards by agreement with other like-minded colleagues?
    Are they 'gold' standards taken from published evidence of best practice?
    Are they 'minimum' standards taken from nationally agreed levels?
    Are they 'average' or 'median' standards for attainment for the profession?
    Are they 'peer' standards (i.e. the level of performance that is acceptable to or attained by your peers)?

•   What data or information will you gather as a baseline?

- When will you start? What is the timetable? Who will do what and when?

- What system do you have for reviewing the results of the audit exercise and comparing performance with pre-set standards? Who will decide and who will make any necessary changes as a result of the exercise?

- How do you compare with your peers, as individuals or other practices?

- What interventions or changes in services or practice will you introduce if your performance does not reach the standards that you have set? What resources will you need for these interventions or changes?

- What specific outcomes do you expect from introducing the intervention(s) or change(s)?

- How will you measure the outcomes?

- How will you demonstrate any improvements or changes from the baseline arising from the intervention(s)?

- When and how will you re-audit?

Significant event audit

Significant events are those that can be used to gain an understanding of the care that an individual or team delivers. They can be based on clinical or non-clinical situations. These can be discussed at practice meetings so as to involve members of the dental team.

This happens in many practices already, but there is pressure on everyone's time, and the lessons to be learned from such incidents are not always documented or disseminated to all members of the team. If discussions take place at practice meetings, then the process is formalised and can be discussed for the maximum benefit of all.

Here are some useful guidelines for such meetings.

1 In general, choose examples where there has been a poor outcome or a 'near miss'.
2 Avoid cases where there may be dento-legal consequences – this is not an appropriate forum for such cases.
3 All members of the team should be involved.
4 Feedback should be constructive, not destructive.
5 The purpose of the meeting is to discuss and explore other ways of dealing with the incident.
6 Appoint a chairperson who has an understanding of the issues.
7 The incident under discussion should be anonymised.
8 The outcomes and proposed changes should be summarised.

9   Remember to be supportive.
10 Agree on the actions to prevent recurrence.

Records of these meetings should be kept confidential, and are another footprint of clinical governance.
   See Chapter 3.

Audit methods

See Chapter 3.

Quality and audit

Quality may be subdivided into eight components as follows:

1   equity
2   access
3   acceptability and responsiveness
4   appropriateness
5   communication
6   continuity
7   effectiveness
8   efficiency.[3]

You might use a matrix as a way of ordering your approach to auditing a particular topic,[4] with eight aspects of quality on the vertical axis, against structure, process and outcome on the horizontal axis. In this way you can generate up to 24 aspects of a particular topic. You might then focus on several aspects in order to look at the quality of patient care or services from various angles.

Quality assurance

Quality assurance consists of quality measurement and quality improvement. Quality assurance has been defined as 'the measurement of actual quality of care against pre-established standards, followed by the implementation of corrective actions to achieve those standards'.[5,6] Quality assurance includes clinical audit, the quality of non-clinical components of services and the practising environment. It is now a Terms of Service requirement for dentists practising in the GDS to have in place a practice-based quality assurance system and to ensure that all members of the dental team participate in the process.

   Continuous quality improvement and total quality management are both umbrella terms which have become devalued over time by their multiple interpretations.

Many health authorities (as they were then) have piloted quality initiatives for general medical practitioners, but initiatives involving dental practices have tended to be restricted to what has been included in the practice visit programme.

Working from what has already been done for medical practitioners, it is likely that any initiatives proposed for dental practices will follow a similar model. Many of the initiatives are based on developing self-assessment tools which rely on a number of indicators of quality.

- *Minimum-level* indicators, many of which are already included in practice visit check-lists because they relate to statutory requirements, are something that every practice is expected to achieve.
- *Desirable-level* indicators relate to examples of good practice, and a practice may have examples of these in specific areas.

A model developed by Northamptonshire Health Authority reviews these indicators under the following six headings:

1 relationships with patients
2 management of risks
3 physical resources
4 staff
5 teamwork
6 practice development and quality management.

When looked at closely, GDPs will recognise these as essential components of running a viable practice from a business point of view.

Another approach has been developed by Bedfordshire Health Authority, which also uses an incremental approach. Its framework is divided into three sections.

- Section I is concerned with essential standards with which practices must comply. These relate to health and safety legislation and employment law.
- Section II contains good practice standards, which many practices will already be meeting.
- Section III focuses on desirable standards which practices can aspire to achieve.

Whatever models are being developed in your locality, the trend is clearly towards a hierarchical approach to looking at quality in general dental practice, and whatever model is being developed, the contents of the final package will be very similar even if the structure may vary.

It should be noted that the development and use of indicators to determine or measure the quality of care is not necessarily an accurate reflection of a high-quality service. The challenge of assessing quality requires an integration of those indicators and their further development to yield meaningful and reliable measures.

This is not an easy task, and it may be that Albert Einstein was right when he made the observation that 'not everything that counts can be counted, and not everything that can be counted counts'.

Audit of a service in the practice

Just as with clinical audit, you must be sure that spending time reviewing the quality of a particular service in the practice is worthwhile. This means that your audit programme must concern an important aspect of your work that crops up sufficiently frequently to justify the effort spent on the audit.

You might audit any of the following:

- the range of services provided in other practices (e.g. specialist services)
- the appropriateness of the services provided – the extent to which services are geared to meeting local needs
- the accessibility of services – where they are located, opening times, internal accessibility to surgeries
- patient information leaflets – type, options for non-English speakers
- publicity – the extent to which the public are aware of the type and availability of services
- skill mix – staffing levels and maximising the potential of PCDs
- training of staff – working within their competencies, sufficient opportunities for continuing professional development
- good employer practices for staff – regular appraisal, regard for health of staff at work, good communication with staff at all levels.

The concept of looking at care in terms of structure, process and outcome has been developed by Maxwell[3] to include aspects of service quality. These are summarised in Table M9.1.

Table M9.1   Assessing different aspects of service quality[3]

Aspect of quality	Questions to ask yourself to help you to assess quality
Effectiveness	Is the treatment provided the best from a technical perspective? Are the materials used the best available for the purpose? What is the evidence to support your intervention? What is the overall result of the treatment?
Acceptability	What does the patient think of the treatment? Was care provided with empathy? How did the patient rate the experience? How do you rate the environment in which it was provided?
Efficiency	Was the care provided in such a way as to achieve maximum benefit for a given and required level of input? How did the cost of providing the care compare with a comparable practice?
Access	Are your patients able to receive care and treatment when they require it? Are there any barriers to care (e.g. waiting times, availability of NHS, cost)?
Equity	Was a particular patient or group of patients treated fairly in comparison with others? Are any particular groups disadvantaged for socio-economic or other reasons?
Relevance	Is the overall pattern and balance of care the best that can be achieved within current constraints of cost, knowledge and technology?

Evaluation of audit

Evaluate your audit work to ensure that the investment of time and effort was worthwhile. You might assess whether:

- everyone participated in the actual audit measuring their performance
- everyone supported and adhered to any changes that were made as a result of audit
- the proposed changes were implemented
- any training needs that were identified were addressed
- any further audits were indicated, and if so whether they were undertaken
- the topic that was audited was important enough to have justified the effort and cost involved
- the method used was appropriate for the purpose of the audit
- the quality of patient care improved
- acceptable outcomes were used to measure any interventions or changes to patient care.

Evaluation of a service

Setting up evaluation of a new service change or model of delivery is complicated by the fact that the outcome may be dependent on many factors other than your own initiative. Sometimes the results may not be immediately obvious and will take time to work through.

Some ways of incorporating evaluation into your everyday work might include the following:

- performance management – to check that the project or service fulfils predetermined criteria of achievement
- external review – undertaken by an independent expert
- internal review – undertaken by members of the project or service providers themselves
- peer review – undertaken by peers in your field.

Alternatively, you might evaluate your initiative or service by assessing the performance or achievement of one or more of the following: activity, personnel, provision of service, practice structure, objectives.

Some ideas on who should do what to apply audit and evaluation in your practice

The GDP

- Advocate audit as a useful tool for the practice team.
- Evaluate your performance and that of the team routinely.

- Make resources available for undertaking audit as necessary.
- Adhere to any changes resulting from the audit as agreed by the primary care team.

The practice manager

- Organise audit so that it is a systematic activity.
- Feed back results of audits to other staff.
- Arrange to undertake audits in parallel with other practices so that you can compare results with your peers in similar settings.
- Discuss the outcomes of the audit with others in the primary care team to gain their ownership of any changes that result.

The dental nurse

- Incorporate audit into your routine work.
- Use a variety of audit methods.
- Suggest topics for future audits when clinical problems crop up.

The receptionist

- Help by gathering data during audit activities.
- Reinforce changes by reminding others about new systems.
- Report problems for patients accessing care that may be appropriate to audit.

Other team members

- Join in any audit activities in the practice at all stages.

References

1 Irvine D and Irvine S (eds) (1991) *Making Sense of Audit*. Radcliffe Medical Press, Oxford. Out of print.

2 Donabedian A (1966) Evaluating the quality of medical care. *Milbank Mem Fund Q.* **44**: 166–204.

3 Maxwell R (1984) Quality assessment in healthcare. *BMJ.* **288**: 1470–2.

4 Firth-Cozens J (1993) *Audit in Mental Health Services*. LEA, Hove.

5 Vuori H (1989) Research needs in quality assurance. *Qual Assur Health Care.* **1**: 147–59.

6 Walshe K and Coles J (1993) *Evaluating Audit. Developing a framework.* CASPE Research, London.

Action plan. Module 9: audit and evaluation

Today's date: ....   Action plan to be completed by: ....

Tackled by	Identify need/assess problem	Plan of action: what will you do?/by when?
Individual – you		
Practice team – you and your colleagues		
Organisation – your practice		

Evaluation: audit and evaluation

Complete an evaluation of progress by ....

Level of evaluation: perspective or work done on this component by	The need or problem	Outcome: what have you achieved?	Who was involved in doing it?	Evaluated: • by whom? • when? • what method was used?
Individual – you				
Practice team – you and your colleagues				
Organisation – your practice				

Record of your learning about 'audit and evaluation'

Write in topic, date, time spent and type of learning activity

	Activity 1	Activity 2	Activity 3	Activity 4
In-house formal learning				
External courses				
Informal and personal				
Qualifications and/or experience gained				

MODULE 10

Meaningful patient involvement

You must be sincere about wanting to involve patients in making decisions about their own care or about the facilities at the practice for such an exercise to be successful.

Real consultation involves a shift of power. Until you are ready for that, any patient involvement in decision making will be a token event. If people feel that their opinions matter and their views are valued and incorporated in the decisions that are made, they will be more likely to co-operate again in the future.

Patient involvement may occur at three levels:

1 for individual patients about their own care
2 about the range and quality of services on offer for patients
3 in planning and organising practice development.

The phrase 'patient involvement' is often used in clinical governance and should be taken to mean individual involvement as a user or patient or, in the case of the big picture, public involvement that includes the processes of consultation and participation. Your strategic health authority/primary care trust will be more involved in the latter than you will.

Advantages of patient involvement

Involving people in making decisions about the services that they receive increases their ownership and gives them more understanding of how the practice operates. This idea of ownership is important. For example, consider the choice of wording that is used in practice information leaflets. Many use the phrase 'Welcome to *our* practice', but some have altered the perspective dramatically by changing just one letter and saying 'Welcome to *your* practice'.

With regard to the big picture, the NHS Executive regards user and public participation as an important priority for all primary care trusts. This approach has been described as 'a test of maturity and openness of the NHS'.[1]

The NHS Executive[2] believes that:

• services are more likely to be appropriate and effective if they are based on needs identified together with users (and the public)

- users are seeking more openness and accountability
- patients want more information about their health condition, treatment and care
- involving patients in their own care may improve healthcare outcomes and increase patient satisfaction
- patients need access to reliable and relevant information in order to be able to assess clinical effectiveness themselves.

Patient involvement depends on people listening and being willing to respond to the views obtained if action is to result.

In the introduction to this book, it was emphasised that the themes of clinical governance are very similar to the tenets of sound business management. The central role of the customer has been emphasised by many business writers and fits well with the principles of clinical governance. Successful business practice puts the customer first and recognises that:[3]

- service quality is relative, not absolute
- it is determined by the customer, not by the service provider
- it varies from one customer to another
- service quality can be enhanced both by meeting or exceeding customers' expectations and by taking steps to control such expectations.

It is unlikely that all patients have the knowledge and the depth of understanding of clinical dentistry necessary to measure the quality of the treatment, but they can almost certainly measure the 'service' elements associated with its provision. The emphasis on a 'patient-centred' service is therefore entirely consistent with the business objectives of a customer-focused practice.

It has also been suggested that the issues involved are far more complex than the current rhetoric implies, and that the emphasis on involving patients has more to do with raising awareness than with policy forming and prioritisation.[4]

Disadvantages of patient involvement

The general consensus is that patient involvement in decision making is a good thing,[5] but GDPs will be aware of situations that can arise when patient empowerment in clinical decision making causes ethical conflict. For example, a patient may not perceive the need for root canal therapy on a non-vital tooth because there is no pain, or they may choose to ignore advice about treating a carious lesion because the tooth is asymptomatic.

This mechanism of patient-led decision making can also operate in the opposite direction. For example, a patient may insist on cosmetic dentistry which, whilst it may satisfy the patient's desires, may leave the clinician with an ethical dilemma if it is the clinician's view that the procedure is too invasive to be justified for cosmetic reasons alone. (The distinction is made here that cosmetic dentistry differs from aesthetic dentistry in that the latter includes a functional element to the decision-making process.) This is a scenario that more and more clinicians are dealing with as the public becomes more aware of and better informed about aesthetic solutions.

Patient expectations

What should patients expect from their healthcare? It has been suggested that the key elements are as follows:[6]

- access – patient care whenever it is needed. This includes access to the Internet and telephone-based services for advice
- personalised – patients should be treated as individuals, and should be offered choices and have an opportunity to indicate their preferences
- control – the system can take control, but only if the patient gives their consent for this
- information – you can know what you wish to know; your clinical records are yours
- science – a right to have care based on the best available scientific knowledge
- safety – patients should not be harmed in their environment
- transparency – confidentiality is assured, but patients will have access to anything and everything about their care and treatment that they wish
- anticipation – pro-active help by anticipating patient needs, which goes beyond mere reactive care
- value – care should not waste the patient's time and money
- co-operation – teams that provide care will co-ordinate efforts to create a seamless experience.

Studies that have investigated patient satisfaction with dental care have identified five generic themes:

1 technical competence
2 interpersonal factors
3 convenience
4 costs
5 facilities.

The results of many surveys have been shown to be contradictory,[7] and this has been partly attributed to a variety of demographic variables, including the following:

- *age* – patients over the age of 60 years tend to be more satisfied with their dental care than younger patients, but less satisfied with the communication process[8]
- *gender* – women express greater levels of satisfaction with dental care than men, perhaps due to their greater exposure to the service, which in turn could have a moderating effect on their expectations[9]
- *economic status* – patients from low-income groups have different attitudes to their dental health and seek care less frequently

- *previous dental experiences* – patients whose previous experience of their dentist has been positive report higher levels of satisfaction. They will forgive the occasional episode of poor performance, attributing this to 'uncontrollable or sporadic elements'[10]
- *regular vs. irregular attendance* – some studies have indicated no difference between the two groups, but others have suggested that there is a positive correlation between frequency of attendance and satisfaction
- *dental anxiety* – it has been shown that patients who exhibit high levels of anxiety tend to be more dissatisfied with their care than their non-anxious counterparts.

The impact of the Health and Social Care Bill

The Health and Social Care Bill has been described as 'legislative machinery that allows the Government to take forward some of the reforms it outlined in the NHS plan published in July 2000 – a plan to "modernise and rebuild" the health service and "reshape" the NHS from the patient's point of view'.[11]

The Bill has added statutory weight to modernise patient representation. Under the terms of the Bill:

1   all NHS trusts, including primary care groups and primary care trusts, will have to ask patients and carers for their views on the services that they have received. Every local NHS organisation will be required to publish an annual patient prospectus, which reports the views received from patients and any action taken as a result

2   a patient advocacy and liaison service (PALS) is to be established in every trust. The Bill signalled the abolition of community health councils (CHCs), which were first established in 1974 as independent health watchdogs. The PALS will:

- act as an independent facilitator for patients, their carers and their families, with the power to negotiate immediate solutions. Patients can also be referred to external or specialist advocacy services, either if requested to do so, or if the PALS considers that this is appropriate
- provide accurate information on all aspects of the trust to help make contact with the NHS as easy as possible
- show patients how to make a complaint about the services that a trust provides
- act as a gateway for patients, their carers and their families who wish to become involved in shaping the NHS.

3   a patients' forum will be established in every trust and the forum will elect a representative on to the trust board

4   a local patients' council is also envisaged for the district, with members drawn from local trust patients' forums

5   health authorities will also have an independent local advisory forum to advise on local health priorities and to contribute to development of the Health Improvement Programme.

The Bill has been welcomed by those 'who believe that services must be driven by local people responding to local needs – and that genuine partnerships between professionals, managers and local communities represent the only effective way forward for the NHS'.[12]

Planning your method of patient involvement

Don't just do a survey because it seems a good idea or because there is a requirement to do it, or it will end up as a meaningless exercise.

Before you start:

- define the purpose
- be realistic about the magnitude of the planned exercise
- select an appropriate method or several methods, depending on the target population and your resources
- obtain the commitment of everyone who will be affected by the exercise
- frame the method in accordance with your perspective
- write the protocol.

Think about the following:

- why you are considering organising a patient involvement exercise – what is the purpose of the exercise?
- whether the exercise really needs to be done
- what structures you already have in place for undertaking patient involvement exercises that you might use
- agreeing the purpose of the exercise with all of your colleagues at work who will be affected by the undertaking and the outcome of the exercise
- being realistic in your choice of method, depending on whether you have identified resources, and whether your practice and colleagues are supportive.

Inappropriate method(s) will mean that patient involvement activities may well end up wasting time and effort as well as needlessly raising other people's expectations about change.

The variety of qualitative methods that can be employed to gather information and views from patients and the general public include the following:

- questionnaires
- focus groups – discussion groups
- interviews
- special-interest patient groups

- consensus events or activities – Delphi surveys, nominal groups, consensus development conferences
- informal feedback from patients – in-house systems such as suggestions boxes, complaints, etc.

Your choice of method is likely to be limited by practical considerations, and you could save time, effort and error by using a method that someone else has already tried and tested for the same purpose in similar circumstances, such as a validated questionnaire or a published interview schedule.

From a practical point of view, most GDPs will probably opt for one or more of the following:

1   questionnaires
2   interviews
3   informal feedback – suggestions box.

Is it worthwhile?

The most important stage of a patient involvement or consultation exercise is listening to the views obtained and responding appropriately.

Your findings are more likely to be implemented if the whole exercise is part of a wider practice development plan, and if the project is 'owned' by the team on whom the results will impact, rather than being the hobbyhorse of one or two people.

When deciding whether the effort and expense was worth it, consider the following:

- whether the information was already available from other sources
- the appropriateness of the costs of the consultation process – were they in proportion to the purpose and the outcomes?
- whether the source of the resources used was appropriate for the purpose and outcomes of the consultation/survey
- the extent to which the results of the consultation/survey were applicable to other groups of people, populations, settings or circumstances, so that you get extra value for the work you have done.

The costs and effort of patient involvement and consultation exercises are wasted if maximum use is not made of the findings. Barriers to change are well known, and you should anticipate some problems in applying the results.[13]

Example 1

If you just ask patients for their views about the services you offer, the information that they give you will provide you with pointers about changes you might consider. Such an exercise in a practice drew the following comments from a variety of patients and relatives who were quizzed at random.

What are the good points about the services provided at this practice?

- 'Easy to talk to.'
- 'Surgery hours are good – very convenient for me.'
- 'The nurses are really helpful and friendly.'
- 'My dentist is brilliant – always tells me everything in layman's terms so I know what's going on.'

What areas are less satisfactory?

- 'Sometimes kept waiting when dentist runs late.'
- 'The magazines are boring. I'm not interested in violins …'
- 'I don't always understand the charges for treatment.'
- 'Sometimes I would like more information about the treatment I am having.'
- 'The waiting-room seats are too low for me.'

Example 2

A survey commissioned by the British Dental Association in 1998 sought to identify what the general public wants from a general dental service.[14] The study involved patient focus groups in different parts of the country, telephone interviews with GDPs, and postal surveys of a number of community health councils. The salient observations were as follows:

- Patients were confused about dental charges, especially the NHS/private mix.
- Patient focus groups felt strongly that charges should be prominently displayed.
- Concerns were expressed about the fee-per-item basis of the dentist's income.
- Cost was identified as a prohibitive factor.
- Concerns were raised about the lack of information about transition from NHS to private practice.
- Longer opening hours were needed to accommodate the needs of working people, as well as a no-appointment-necessary system.
- Dentists should keep up to date and work from an evidence base.
- There was a perception that there was a lack of redress for substandard dental work.
- More emphasis should be placed on prevention and on looking after children's dental health.

- There should be improved service provision for phobic dental patients.
- More comfortable waiting-rooms were needed.

Many of the conclusions drawn from this survey bear a remarkable similarity to the *Barriers to the Receipt of Dental Care Report*, published over 10 years earlier.[15]

Interpersonal skills

At the centre of patient involvement lies the communication process. GDPs must assess and develop the communication skills of all members of the team if patients are to become involved in a meaningful way. Patients have described what they understand by communication skills through a questionnaire. They identified ten aspects of inter-personal skills that were important to them:

1 being greeted warmly
2 being listened to
3 clear explanations
4 reassurance
5 showing confidence
6 being able to express concerns and fears
7 being respected
8 having enough time during the visit
9 consideration of their personal context
10 concern for the patient as a person.

This list could be used as a guide to assessing the quality of the interpersonal relationships that exist between members of your team and your patients, and it may also provide you with an outline action plan on how to improve those core skills.

Charter Mark

The national Charter Mark award was established to help public sector organisations to make real improvements in the delivery of services, from the point of view of the people who matter the most, namely the 'customers'.

There are ten Charter Mark criteria, reference to which may be useful in creating a more market-orientated NHS. They are listed below.

Criterion 1: Set standards

Set clear standards of service that users can expect, and monitor and review performance and publish the results, following independent validation, wherever possible.

Criterion 2: Be open and provide full information

Be open, and communicate clearly and effectively in plain language to help people using public services. Also provide full information about services, their cost and how well they perform.

Criterion 3: Consult and involve

Consult and involve current and potential users of public services as well as those who work in them, and use their views to improve the service provided.

Criterion 4: Encourage access and the promotion of choice

Make services easily available to everyone who needs them, including using new technology to the full, and offering choice wherever possible.

Criterion 5: Treat all fairly

Treat all people fairly, respect their privacy and dignity, be helpful and courteous, and pay particular attention to those with special needs.

Criterion 6: Put things right when they go wrong

Put things right quickly and effectively, learn from complaints, and have a clear, well-publicised and easy-to-use complaints procedure, with independent review wherever possible.

Criterion 7: Use resources effectively

Use resources effectively to provide best value for taxpayers and users.

Criterion 8: Innovate and improve

Always look for ways to improve the services and facilities offered, particularly the use of new technology.

Criterion 9: Work with other providers

Work with other providers to ensure that services are simple to use, effective and co-ordinated, and deliver a better service to the user.

Criterion 10: Provide user satisfaction

Show that your users are satisfied with the quality of service that they are receiving.

These criteria were used in one study designed to assess whether patients themselves considered the criteria to be important in the provision of good-quality dental services.[16] The study concluded that although patients are interested in 'information on standards, performance and complaints, there is considerable disinterest in organisational and financial dimensions'.

Focus Awards

The Focus Award scheme is a joint initiative by the Department of Health and the British Dental Association, and reflects the current thinking on meaningful patient involvement. The first Focus Awards for patient-focused innovations in dentistry were presented in October 2001. The categories under which a practice may be nominated for these awards are as follows:

- patients' experiences when contacting the practice
- patients' experiences whilst in the reception or waiting area
- patients' experiences during clinical treatment
- general communication with patients
- any other significant patient-focused innovation.

At the time of writing, this award scheme is about to enter its second year.

Showing your commitment

Your commitment to involving patients can be summarised in your practice statement about quality assurance in your practice. An example is shown below, and is reproduced by kind permission of Andrew Keetley of the Family Dental Practice in Kirk Hallam.

QUALITY ASSURANCE SYSTEMS AT THIS PRACTICE

1   Our practice aims to provide dental care of a consistent quality, for all our patients. We have management systems to help us, and which define each practice member's responsibilities when looking after you.
2   In proposing treatment, we will take into account your own wishes. We will explain options, where appropriate, and costs, so that you can make an informed choice. We will always explain what we are doing.
3   We will do all we can to look after your general health. We will ask you about your general health, and about any medicines being taken. This helps us treat you safely. We keep all information about you confidential.
4   Contamination control is also essential to the safety of our patients. Every practice member receives training in practice systems for contamination control.
5   We screen all patients for mouth cancer at routine check-ups. We ask patients about tobacco and alcohol use because they increase your oral cancer risk.

6 Practice working methods are reviewed regularly at meetings of all staff. We encourage all staff to make suggestions for improving the care we give patients.
7 We regularly ask patients for their views on our services. We have systems for dealing promptly with patient complaints and for ensuring that lessons are learned from any mistakes we make.
8 All dentists in the practice take part in continuing professional education, meeting the General Dental Council's requirements. We aim to keep up to date with current thinking on all aspects of general dentistry, including preventive care, which reduces your need for treatment.
9 All staff joining the practice are given training in practice-wide procedures. Once a year there is an individual review of training needs for everyone in the practice.
10 All members of the practice know of the need to ensure that dentists are working safely. In the unlikely event that a dentist in this practice becomes unfit to practise, we have systems to ensure that concerns are investigated and, if necessary, acted upon.

Some ideas on who should do what to establish meaningful involvement of patients in your practice

The GDP

- Welcome unsolicited patient views and act on suggestions.
- Set up meaningful patient involvement systems; incorporate patient input into decision making (e.g. into the practice's business plan).
- Learn more about various methods of public consultation in order to understand which may be appropriate in given situations.

The practice manager

- Organise various methods of patient involvement and consultation.
- Consider setting up a panel of patients drawn from patients of the practice – for patients to respond with their views.
- Provide patients with good information about practice systems.
- Find out whether you can co-ordinate your activities with other initiatives involving the strategic health authority or primary care trust.

The dental nurse

- Suggest important topics on which the practice might consult.

- Participate in consultation exercises by administering a short questionnaire to a sample of patients.
- Prepare patient literature giving information about various clinical conditions; encourage questions.

The receptionist

- Administer the suggestions box; empty it out regularly and pass on suggestions to the practice manager.
- Record every comment and suggestion from patients so that the practice can look for trends.
- Help with any data collection, such as administering surveys.

References

1   Lugon M and Scally G (2000) *Clin Gov Bull.* **1**(1): 1.

2   NHS Executive (1997) *Priorities and Planning Guidelines for the NHS: medium-term priorities.* The Stationery Office, London.

3   Miller JA (1977) Studying satisfaction, modifying models, eliciting expectations, posing problems and making meaningful measurements. In: HK Hunt (ed.) *Conceptualisation and Making Meaningful Measurements.* Marketing Science Institute, Cambridge, MA.

4   Milewa T (1997) Community participation and healthcare priorities: reflections on policy, theatre and reality in Britain. *Health Prom Int.* **12**: 161–8.

5   Gibbons DE, Gelbier S and Newton T (2000) The oral health of minority ethnic groups in contemporary Britain: a case study of the South Thames Region. GKT Dental Institute, London.

6   Institute of Medicine Committee (2001) *Crossing the Quality Chasm: a new health system for the 21st century.* IOM, Washington DC.

7   Newsome PRH and Wright GH (1992) A review of patient satisfaction. *Br Dent J.* **186**: 166–70.

8   Stege P, Handleman S, Baric J and Espekand M (1986) Satisfaction of the older patient with dental care. *Gerodontics.* **2**: 171–4.

9   Gopalakrishna P and Mummalaneni V (1993) Influencing satisfaction for dental services. *J Health Care Market.* **13**: 16–22.

10 Clow K, Fischer A and O'Bryan D (1995) Patient expectations of dental services. *J Health Care Market.* **15**: 23–31.

11 Butler P (2001) www.societyguardian.co.uk

12 Dr Michael Dixon. NHS Alliance Chairman press comment. 9 November 2001.

13 Dunning M, Abi-Aad G, Gilbert D *et al.* (1999) *Experience, Evidence and Everyday Practice.* King's Fund, London.

14 Land T (2000) What patients think of dental services. *Br Dent J.* **189**: 21–4.

15 Finch H (1987) *Barriers to the Receipt of Dental Care: a qualitative research study.* London Social and Community Planning Research, London.

16 Crossley ML, Blinkhorn A and Cox M (2001) What do our patients really want from us? Investigating the patient's perceptions of the validity of the Charter Mark criteria. *Br Dent J.* **190**: 602–6.

Action plan. Module 10: meaningful patient involvement

Today's date: ....   Action plan to be completed by: ....

Tackled by	Identify need/assess problem	Plan of action: what will you do?/by when?
Individual – you		
Practice team – you and your colleagues		
Organisation – your practice		

Evaluation: meaningful patient involvement

Complete an evaluation of progress by ....

Level of evaluation: perspective or work done on this component by	The need or problem	Outcome: what have you achieved?	Who was involved in doing it?	Evaluated: • by whom? • when? • what method was used?
Individual – you				
Practice team – you and your colleagues				
Organisation – your practice				

Record of your learning about 'meaningful patient involvement'

Write in topic, date, time spent and type of learning activity

	Activity 1	Activity 2	Activity 3	Activity 4
In-house formal learning				
External courses				
Informal and personal				
Qualifications and/or experience gained				

MODULE 11

Health promotion

Different approaches to health promotion[1] include the following:

- medical and preventative behaviour change
- educational approaches
- empowerment of the individual
- social change.

You need to consider how you can inform patients about health risks and how you can help patients to change their behaviour.

Table M11.1 summarises one model for health education.[2]

Table M11.1 Model for health education

1 Health persuasion	Interventions by professionals, aimed at individuals (e.g. advice to stop smoking or to take exercise)
2 Legislative action	Intervention by professionals, aimed at communities (e.g. lobbying for legal changes in school sex education programmes)
3 Personal counselling	Led by individual need, performed by professionals (e.g. professionals helping an individual choose treatments when options are available)
4 Community action	Led by community needs, performed by professionals (e.g. professionals helping a group to lobby for a local resource)

Targeting

Broadly speaking there are two approaches. You can target whole populations (e.g. giving advice on the prevention of dental diseases to everyone you see), or you can target high-risk groups of patients.

The scientific approach can be criticised for ignoring the social and environmental aspects of disease. It tends to encourage dependence on scientific knowledge and can remove health decisions from individuals. Health professionals need to develop strategies to encourage individual action (another example of patient empowerment) and reduce attitudes of coercion or blame.

Health promotion can only be effective if patients can access the services available. Workers in the health service will be mainly concerned with activities 1 and 3 in Table M11.1. They may become involved individually in more community-orientated activities

(2 and 4) on occasion by joining pressure groups, charities or lay organisations as professional advisers, etc.

One of the five short-listed entrants in the recent Department of Health/British Dental Association Focus Award scheme was a practice which offered the services of a smoking cessation adviser as part of its wider obligations to health promotion among its patients.[3]

National initiatives

Mouth Cancer Awareness Week (11–17 November 2001) was an initiative supported by a nationwide publicity campaign. This 'blue-ribbon' campaign was designed to increase awareness among the public of a condition which affects 3800 people in the UK alone each year, with fewer than 50% of those diagnosed surviving five years.[4] Oral cancer kills more people each year than cervical cancer and skin melanoma. It is a sad fact that most cases are diagnosed only after the appearance of symptomatic growths.

The role of the general dental practitioner is to be involved in the following:

- raising awareness of oral cancer
- primary prevention – changing people's behaviour
- secondary prevention – early detection through screening
- tertiary prevention – preventing recurrence in patients who have already been treated for oral cancer.

The British Dental Health Foundation (BDHF) supported the National No Smoking Day on 14 March 2002. The aim of the campaign was to improve public access to advice and information about important oral health issues such as smoking and oral cancer.

National Smile Week is another oral health awareness campaign organised each May by the BDHF as part of its activities to promote dental care to the general public.

These events provide good opportunities for GDPs as far as health promotion initiatives are concerned, because organisations such as the BDHF provide a wide variety of support materials for dental practitioners to use.

Ethical problems

The essential nature of health education is that it is voluntary. If patients attend for advice or treatment for a particular problem, is it right to include opportunistic information gathering in the consultation? Patients may not have given their *full informed consent* to these activities.

Patients may fear that refusal to consent to health promotion activities will affect the way in which you manage the problems with which they have attended. You have an extra responsibility if you involve patients in these activities. *See* the Checklist on page 181.

People with disabilities

Access to health promotion activities is often difficult for those with physical handicaps, visual or hearing impairment, etc. Think about how to provide informational materials other than in traditional leaflet format.

Videos, audio tapes, picture-based formats and role play are all useful tools.

You could also consider how you could take dental health promotion to selected groups, as the community dental service has been doing.

People with learning disabilities have the same right as anyone else to make their own decisions. Just because it takes more time, or the information has to be explained in a different way, the competence of these patients to understand and to make their own decisions must not be underestimated.

Break information into smaller-sized chunks. Use pictures, drawings and models even more than you usually would. Give the patient simple information sheets to take away.

Evaluation of health promotion

Preventive measures are ultimately evaluated by a reduction in dental disease. Shorter-term evaluation, such as an increase in the number of people being offered health promotion activities, has often been used instead. Such enumeration is unable to measure any change in behaviour.

You need to consider what outcomes[5] you might be able to measure and how reliable they might be. Timing of evaluations can be difficult. An immediate post-programme evaluation may not be sustained after six months, or changes may take time to be manifested (*see* Module 9 on Audit and evaluation).

Pitfalls of enumeration

An emphasis on evaluation has led to health promotion activities being based more on what can be measured than on effective measures that are less easily quantified. Results are interpreted differently according to the viewpoint of the receiver of the report.

- A funder of a project may insist on cost-effectiveness.
- A practitioner may be looking for acceptability to the patient.
- Managers may measure success by indicators of increased productivity.
- Patients may want to increase their control over some aspect of their health.

The ideal is to be able to present all of these facets in a report about a health promotion activity. A further difficulty is being sure that the changes measured are due to the health promotion activities rather than to any other external change. Confounding external factors may influence your results.

Evaluation is only worth doing if it will make a difference to what you do next. Interpretation and feedback to those involved must be incorporated into the design. Evaluation is not a simple activity, and it may consume resources that could be employed more constructively. Monitoring of activity may be all that can be achieved, but you should be clear about the differences between monitoring and evaluation.

Advantages of health promotion

- Professionals are perceived by the public to have credibility. For example, a survey by *Health Education* and the Consumers' Association found that 95% of respondents trusted their family doctor and 87% trusted the nurse. Other sources of information were much less trusted. For example, radio and television were trusted by 63% of respondents, and newspapers and magazines by only 25%.
- Local services are more accessible.
- Repeated contact builds up trust and increases opportunities for reinforcing health education messages.
- For patients who attend regularly for an examination before disease becomes established, the opportunities for giving preventive advice are enhanced.
- Adding on to established provision is cheaper than providing new facilities.

Disadvantages of health promotion activities in general dental practice

- Dentists and nurses are often not adequately trained or competent in health promotion activities.
- They should not be involved in activities designed solely to meet the demands of income generation at the expense of meeting demonstrable health needs.
- The value of health checks, regardless of health status, is unclear. There are few screening activities that have benefits clearly based on evidence rather than on hope.
- Those who would benefit most from lifestyle advice are least likely to take up services on offer.
- Those who need to make the greatest lifestyle changes often have environmental constraints, such as poverty or poor housing, which are mainly susceptible to political or community changes.
- The demands of a fee-for-item service are more immediate and leave little time or opportunity for health promotion activities.

Checklist to help you think about health promotion[1]

Central considerations in working for health

- Are you enabling people to direct their own lives?
- Do you respect people's decisions even if they conflict with your own?
- Do you treat people equally?
- Do you work with people on the basis that those who need your help most come first?

Key ethical principles[6]

- Are you doing more good than harm?
- Are you telling the truth and keeping promises?

Consequences of ways of working for health

- Will your actions increase the health of the individual?
- Will your actions increase the health of a particular group?
- Will your actions increase the health of society?
- Will your actions have any effect on your own health?

External consequences of working for health

- Are there any legal considerations?
- Is there a risk attached to the intervention?
- Is this intervention the most effective and efficient action to take?
- How certain is the evidence on which this intervention is based?
- What are the views and wishes of those involved?
- Can I justify my actions in terms of all this evidence?

'Prevention is better than cure' is only true if it is effective and acceptable to both provider and recipient.

Some ideas on who should do what to increase health promotion activities

The GDP

- Incorporate reminders on patient records.

- Identify target groups for health promotion activities.
- Take opportunities to promote health pro-actively, and record what advice has been given.

The practice manager

- Decide who is responsible for what health promotion activities in the practice.
- Support staff in learning best practice.
- Provide time for dental health promotion activities.

The dental nurse

- Innovate new ways of informing people about health.
- Run patient groups.
- Use templates or structured records for recording health promotion activities.

The receptionist

- Invite patients for health promotion activities.
- Publicise practice activities.

The dental hygienist

- Provide relevant educational material.
- Be aware of health promotional activities in the practice.
- Encourage patient participation.

References

1   Naidoo J and Wills J (1994) *Health Promotion: foundations for practice*. Balliere Tindall, London.

2   Beattie A (1991) In: J Gabe, M Calnan and M Bury (eds) *The Sociology of the Health Service*. Routledge, London.

3   68, The Dental Practice and Implant Clinic, Crossgate, Leeds, West Yorkshire.

4   Cancer Research Campaign (CRC) *Cancerstats: Oral – UK*. July 2000.

5   Tones K, Tilford S and Robinson Y (1990) *Health Education: effectiveness and efficiency*. Chapman & Hall, London.

6   Doxiadis S (ed.) (1990) *Ethics in Health Promotion*. John Wiley & Sons, Chichester.

Websites

http://www.wolfson.tvu.ac.uk/learn/links/promo.stm is a useful website with many other links to health promotion information.

Further reading

Pike S and Forster D (1995) *Health Promotion for All*. Churchill Livingstone, Edinburgh.
    This book contains a framework for developing a personal health promotion portfolio.

Action plan. Module 11: health promotion

Today's date: .... Action plan to be completed by: ....

Tackled by	Identify need/assess problem	Plan of action: what will you do?/by when?
Individual – you		
Practice team – you and your colleagues		
Organisation – your practice		

Evaluation: health promotion

Complete an evaluation of progress by ....

Level of evaluation: perspective or work done on this component by	The need or problem	Outcome: what have you achieved?	Who was involved in doing it?	Evaluated: • by whom? • when? • what method was used?
Individual – you				
Practice team – you and your colleagues				
Organisation – your practice				

Record of your learning about 'health promotion'

Write in topic, date, time spent and type of learning activity

	Activity 1	Activity 2	Activity 3	Activity 4
In-house formal learning				
External courses				
Informal and personal				
Qualifications and/or experience gained				

MODULE 12

Risk management

Risk management is an essential element of clinical governance. However, it is a widely misunderstood phrase, and its meaning has tended to reflect the context of its usage. For example, in business and insurance it has reflected the need to promote the interests of the business for its shareholder. In this context it has been defined as:

> 'the identification, measurement, control, financing and transfer of risks which threaten life, property and the continued viability of enterprises'.[1]

In health and safety terms, it relates to the risk of one party being managed by another. In the field of professional indemnity, and particularly where the indemnity provider is a mutual organisation, it implies a co-operative approach with all parties playing an important part.

For the purposes of clinical governance, a useful definition is that risk management is 'a means of reducing the risks of adverse events occurring in organisations by systematically assessing, reviewing and then seeking ways to prevent their occurrence'. Clinical risk management takes place in a clinical setting.

Good organisation and efficient practice systems should reduce the likelihood of mistakes occurring.

Risks may be prevented, avoided, minimised or managed where they cannot be reduced. If things do go wrong, it is important to learn from the experience, and this is a recurring theme within the risk management area of clinical governance.

Principles of risk management

The continuum of risk management can be summarised by a number of guiding principles that fall into one of the following four categories:

- risk awareness
- risk control
- risk containment
- risk transfer.

Risk awareness

This refers to the understanding of those activities and situations that carry a high risk of problems arising. This awareness can be achieved by reference to the following:

1   case studies often reported in the annual reports of the professional indemnity providers
2   discussions during team meetings
3   internal reporting mechanisms for adverse incidents.

It should be noted that not all risks relate to clinical situations.

Risk control

Any activity that involves taking practical steps to avoid or minimise risk is an example of risk control. The use of rubber dam as airway protection during endodontic procedures is a good clinical example. The management of the patient's expectations and therefore the delivery of a satisfactory outcome in relation to those expectations is a good non-clinical example, and it relies heavily on the ability of the dentist and/or team to communicate effectively.

Risk containment

When problems do arise, it is essential to manage the situation with empathy to ensure that the concerns are addressed in-house as much as possible. Part of the strategy for achieving this again relies on effective communication and prompt responses to the patient's concerns. Advice is always available from your defence organisation in this respect.

Risk transfer

In paying their subscriptions to their defence organisation, GDPs transfer the financial component of the risk to the indemnity provider.

Record keeping (also *see* Module 4 on Reliable and accurate data)

Good record keeping is as important as the provision of good dentistry, and is an integral part of the use of reasonable skill and care. It is one of the most important factors in risk management.[2]

The information on the patient's record card should include the following:

•   records of all advice given with regard to alternative treatment plans

- the appropriate consents obtained
- the treatment provided
- preoperative and postoperative advice and warnings given
- unusual sequelae
- medication/drugs prescribed or dispensed
- treatment which the patient was unwilling to undergo
- a record of every visit
- cancelled or failed appointments
- telephone advice given.

The defence organisations are keen to emphasise that poor records make for a poor defence in cases of litigation, and no record means no defence.

You might test out how you fare against the following six recommended stages of good record keeping that reduce the likelihood of mistakes being made or patient care forgotten.

- *Stage 1.* Are the dental records complete and legible? Do all of the team members in the practice who are actively contributing to providing care for the patient have access to the dental records?
- *Stage 2.* Have the notes been summarised so that the pages are in consecutive order, all of the key information is readily available, and any important past and current history has been entered in all of the relevant databases and the practice's review systems?
- *Stage 3.* Are the records stored in such a way (paper and/or computerised records) that they can be readily retrieved for use in a consultation? Is the filing up to date so that all correspondence is available when the patient is under treatment?
- *Stage 4.* Are all contacts entered in the records, including telephone consultations?
- *Stage 5.* Are the medical records stored securely in fireproof cabinets if they are paper based, with access only to those with authority whether they are paper-based or computer records? Are regular back-ups of computer records made, with the back-up disks being stored off the surgery premises?
- *Stage 6.* Are records kept of all referrals sent off? Are all outcomes of such referrals reviewed and acted upon if necessary?

Clinical risk management

Clinical risk management is about what goes wrong during patient care and why, and is concerned with learning lessons from these incidents to ensure that action is taken to prevent recurrence. It is about minimising risk by ensuring that:[3]

- clinical teams are appropriately trained
- individual members of the team are aware of their role and responsibilities
- the environment in which the team operates is safe.

In your practice, you might focus on critical incidents such as instrument separation in endodontics, or lateral perforation during post hole preparation, to explore the different aspects of risk management. The importance of using such incidents has been emphasised in the Government's 1997 White Paper entitled *The New NHS: modern, dependable*.[4]

In order to deliver this part of the clinical governance agenda, your practice should have in place the following:

- a sound clinical risk management process that encourages critical incident reporting
- staff who are aware of it and understand it
- effective claims management.

Risk assessment: health and safety in primary care

An employer's duty[5] is to:

- make the workplace safe and without risks to health – of staff or visiting patients
- ensure that articles and substances are moved, stored and used safely
- provide adequate welfare facilities
- inform, instruct, train and supervise staff as necessary for their health and safety
- keep dust, fumes and noise under control
- ensure that plant and machinery are safe, and that safe systems of work are set and followed
- draw up a health and safety policy statement if there are five or more employees, and make staff aware of the policy and arrangements
- provide adequate first-aid facilities.

Applying clinical governance to health and safety at work

Examples of how you might do this in bite-sized chunks of work are listed below.

- *Confidentiality*: data on staff sickness absence should be kept confidentially, especially if the member of staff is also a patient registered with the practice.
- *Risk management*: anticipate problems by health surveillance looking for common sources of stress for staff, and minimise that stress.
- *Health gain*: safer premises for patients – look for obstacles which might cause patients to trip in the grounds of or within the surgery.
- *Health promotion*: assess staff safety and look for ways to improve safety in the surgery.
- *Research and development*: is there a burning issue you might investigate, such as how practices in your district are sterilising their equipment in main and branch surgeries?

- *Learning culture*: health and safety would be a good topic to discuss as a practice team. You might invite an expert on infection control from the PCT. You could discuss any problems detected by your comprehensive programme on health and safety.
- *Core requirements*: all staff should be aware of the requirement to comply with health and safety law, and the extent to which health and safety law applies to their posts.
- *Managing resources and services*: branch surgeries should meet the requirements of health and safety law in just the same way as the main surgery does.
- *Reliable and accurate data*: keep comprehensive records of checks to equipment, emergency drugs, and shelf-life of materials.
- *Involving patients and the public*: ask a patient to walk around the practice and point out any hazards from their own perspective. Act on any patients' complaints.
- *Evidence-based practice*: find out and apply best practice in minimising and eliminating cross-infection.
- *Audit*: undertake an audit of some aspects of your practice.
- *Accountability*: ensure that systems which comply with the law are in place and applied.
- *Coherent team*: check that everyone is up to date with practice systems and procedures for ensuring health and safety.

Innovation – and risk taking

Innovation involves an element of risk taking and uncertainty. The vision of the primary care model of the future with different types of provision will be threatened if the workforce is not sufficiently flexible and willing to adapt to different ways of working. Retention of staff is very important if the innovation is to succeed, for if staff are not supported in change management, a proportion will leave.

There are a number of risks envisaged by those prophesying how primary care will develop. The vision is not without risks[6] such as the following:

- the potential loss of the 'personal touch' for patients as some primary care is provided via telephone helplines and information technology
- loss of continuity of care as a trade-off with offering patients more convenient and faster access to primary care advice and information
- insufficient capacity in primary care to meet the expanded range of services envisaged
- insufficiently flexible staffing, structures and budgets to achieve innovative models of service delivery whilst retaining uniformly high-quality primary care.

Controlling risk factors

The magnitude of risk is derived from the 'likelihood' and the 'severity' of negative outcomes occurring.[7] When people weigh up a risk and make a conscious decision about whether to take that risk, they:

- identify the possible options
- identify the consequences or outcomes that might follow from each of those options
- evaluate the desirability of each consequence
- estimate the likelihood of each consequence associated with a specific option
- combine these steps to make a decision – taking into account their own preferences and habitual behaviour.

People usually have a reasonable idea of the *relative* risks of various activities and behaviours, although their estimates of the *magnitude* of risks tend to be biased – small probabilities are often overestimated, and large probabilities are often underestimated. However, people may underestimate the risk when they apply relative risks to themselves and their own behaviour. For example, many smokers accept the relationship between smoking tobacco and disease, but do not believe that they personally are at risk.[1] People claim that they are less likely than their peers to suffer harm, which makes it less likely that they will take precautions. Thus if you wish to modify people's behaviour so that they adopt less risky lifestyles, you should not only provide information about risk, but also reinforce your messages by engaging the person in considering the costs and benefits of the behavioural alternatives.[1]

Adverse events/accidents

The following terms may be useful, and are taken from the definitions provided in the Department of Health publication *An Organisation With a Memory*.[8]

- *Adverse healthcare event*: an event or omission arising during clinical care and causing physical or psychological injury to a patient.
- *Error*: the failure to complete a planned action as intended, or the use of an incorrect plan of action to achieve a given aim.
- *Hazard*: anything that can cause harm.
- *Healthcare near miss*: a situation in which an event or omission, or a sequence of events or omissions, arising during clinical care fails to develop further, whether or not as a result of compensating action, thus preventing injury to a patient.
- *Risk*: the likelihood (high or low) that someone or something will be harmed by a hazard, multiplied by the severity of the potential harm.
- *System*: a set of interdependent elements that interact to achieve a common aim. These elements may be both human and non-human (equipment, technologies, etc.).

About 75% of accidents are caused by human beings, but the increasing sophistication and complexity of equipment are known to be an increasing source of accidents.

Strategy

An expert group under the chairmanship of the Chief Medical Officer has now published its report,[8] which examines the strengths and weaknesses of the NHS systems for learning from adverse events. The report 'sets out to review what we know about the scale and nature of serious failures in NHS healthcare, to examine the extent to which the NHS has the capacity to learn from such failures when they do occur, and to recommend measures which could help to ensure that the likelihood of repeated failures is minimised in the future'.

The report noted that there was wide variation in the interpretation of adverse events, and not all staff understood the definition of an adverse event.

The report made a number of recommendations, which provide us with a useful framework for a risk management strategy. It noted that there are four key areas that must be addressed:

1   unified mechanisms for reporting and analysis when things go wrong
2   a more open culture, in which errors or service failures can be reported and discussed
3   mechanisms for ensuring that, where lessons are identified, the necessary changes are put into practice
4   a much wider appreciation of the value of the system approach in preventing, analysing and learning from errors.

GDPs can use this approach to develop their own risk management strategy in general practice.

To err is human

Human beings make mistakes. Mistakes in general dental practice affect clinical outcomes for the patient, and can cost reputations and money. Years of sustained effort in practice building can be undone by a handful of adverse incidents.

So-called unsafe acts have been classified into two groups:

1   errors
2   violations.

Errors are usually attributed to either of the following:

1   *attentional slippage*, which occurs when there is an unintended deviation from a sound treatment plan
2   *mistakes*, where a clinical action may well follow a treatment plan, but it is the plan which deviates from the path which would have produced the desired outcome. This can be subdivided into two groups:

   •   *rule-based mistakes*, where a clinician encounters a familiar problem but applies the wrong solution

- *knowledge-based mistakes,* where a clinician encounters a situation for which they have received inadequate training to apply a rule-based solution.

Studies have been conducted to try to quantify error probability. It has been suggested that performing a totally new task with little idea of the possible outcomes carries an error probability of 0.75. At the other end of the spectrum, the execution of a highly familiar task by a competent and experienced practitioner carries an error probability of 0.0005. This means that the error is likely to occur five times in 10 000 discrete events.

Error probability has been shown to be affected by a number of error-producing conditions.

In practical terms, these conditions can be banded into the following groups:

1   high workload (sometimes known as quantitative overload)
2   inadequate knowledge and skills (sometimes known as qualitative overload)
3   inadequate supervision
4   stressful working environment
5   mental state (boredom and fatigue are two common examples)
6   management of change.

A practice-based risk management calls for an understanding of these broad categories. Measures should be put in place to limit both the frequency and the probability of error.

Violations, on the other hand, arise when there is a deliberate or unrecognised deviation from a regulated code of practice.

Violations can lead to various penalties, including the following:

1   the imposition of direct penalties – such as disciplinary action if a dentist is found in breach of their Terms of Service
2   restrictions or conditional practising arrangements which can restrict a practitioner's ability to provide care and treatment without first seeking the necessary authority (e.g. prior approval criteria which have been imposed by the Dental Practice Board)
3   suspension or erasure imposed by the General Dental Council in cases where it has been deemed that the violation amounts to serious professional misconduct.

Factors that seem to promote violations are less well understood and more difficult to analyse. Violation-producing conditions include the following:

- poor supervision and control
- group norms condoning violations
- misperception of hazards
- a macho culture which encourages risk taking
- low self-esteem
- perceived licence to bend rules
- ambiguous rules.

Many violations also tend to be based on the principle of risk reward. Random checking to ensure that dentists are complying with the rules and regulations of the system within which they work is based on small-number sampling, and the perception may be that such sampling will not always reveal occasional violations.

Active failure and latent failure

These are usually due to a combination of individual and organisational factors.

Human error is commonly blamed for failures because it is often the most readily identifiable factor.[8] Interestingly, Mr Justice Sheen's report into the tragic capsizing of the *Herald of Free Enterprise* in 1987 highlighted this by drawing attention to the subtle but real difference between *active human failures* and *latent human failures*. The member of the crew who failed to shut the bow doors provides an example of *active* failure, and the inadequate organisational policies (*latent* failures) created an environment in which active failures were more likely to occur.

Active failures are unsafe acts committed by people who carry responsibility for care. The errors and violations described earlier are examples.

Latent conditions are organisational flaws – latent conditions with the potential to cause failure. They can be identified, isolated and removed before they lead to an adverse event.

One model of accident causation, popular in aviation and the nuclear industry, is known as the Swiss Cheese Model of accident causation (*see* Figure M12.1).

The dangers present when the holes in the model (due to active and latent factors) align to create a pathway to accident causation when hazards lead to resultant losses. The trick is to create systems and barriers which minimise the risk of 'hole alignment' and block the path of accident causation. The more slices of cheese we have, the lower the likelihood that something catastrophic will occur. Well-thought-out systems, processes, protocols and guidelines which are the very essence of practice management should combine to form part of the risk management strategy for the practice.

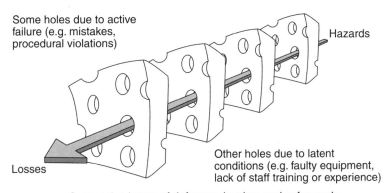

Figure M12.1   The 'Swiss cheese' model of accident causation.[9]

Useful tips

In one report, two leading authorities on risk management were asked for their five top tips on risk management. A summary of their advice is given below.

David Hewett's tips[12.1]

- Value and respect the members of your team. Healthcare staff are often devastated when something goes wrong – there is no need to reiterate what has happened.
- Move away from 'naming and shaming'. Errors often occur because of system break-down, which in turn puts team members in situations where errors and violations are more likely to occur.
- Support your team members – do not exclude them. Suspension and exclusion are often perceived in the wrong way.
- The investigation of the incident should be fair and open. Follow up change by monitoring the situation.
- Be aware of risk at every level of the organisation.

Keith Haynes' tips[12.2]

- Recognise and promote risk management as a tool to improve the quality of services provided.
- Start by conducting a risk assessment. Sit the team down and identify and rate the risks, and the discussions of the team can often form part of your quality-improvement agenda.
- Make risk management a regular feature of your work routine. Ensure that you have regular team meetings to discuss the issues.
- Remember to review entire systems rather than focus on individual roles. Remember that when things go wrong, the systems often break down, so it is about systems rather than individuals.
- Remember that effective risk management is about the quality of care that you provide.

In recent studies it has been shown that as many as 80% of adverse events were systems related rather than involving a person. Of course people matter, but remember to place them in an environment where the systems help them and do not hinder them. How will you know whether this is the case? Try asking them. In a word, communicate!

Relative risk is deduced by comparing the effects of being 'highly' exposed to the risk factor with the effects of being 'slightly' or not at all exposed to that factor. There is a proportional change in the risk of an outcome for a given change in the level of the risk factor.

[12.1]David Hewett, Chairman of the Association of Litigation and Risk Management (ALARM).

[12.2]Keith Haynes, Head of Risk Management Services, Medical Protection Society, Leeds.

Some ideas on who should do what to put risk management into practice

The GDP

- Be clear what employer's responsibilities for health and safety you are delegating to the practice manager.
- Provide resources so that the practice complies with health and safety laws.
- Recognise and anticipate risks, and either eliminate, avoid or minimise them.
- Adhere to practice systems and procedures designed to manage risk.

The practice manager

- Help to establish policies for risk management.
- Monitor policies for risk management.
- Carry out risk reduction programmes in the practice.
- Establish good communication systems in the practice to alert staff about risks.

The dental nurse

- Tend the equipment in the surgery to minimise risks.
- Ensure that it operates efficiently by adhering closely to the maintenance programme, including start-up and shut-down procedures.
- Store dangerous substances in a secure way.
- Help to ensure patient compliance with safety (e.g. wearing protective spectacles, etc.).

The receptionist

- Contribute to any monitoring procedures to detect or review risks.
- Respond to any personal alarm system indicating that a staff member feels their safety is being threatened.

References

1   Institute of Risk Management (1991) *Student Handbook*. Institute of Risk Management, London.

2   *Essentials of Risk Management*. Dental Protection Ltd. Member publication.

3   Lugon M and Scally G (2000) Editorial. *Clin Gov Bull*. **1**(2): 1–2.

4   Department of Health (1997) *The New NHS: modern, dependable.* The Stationery Office, London.

5   Higson N (1996) *Risk Management. Health and safety in primary care.* Butterworth-Heinemann, Oxford.

6   Coffey T, Boersma G, Smith L and Wallace P (1999) *Visions of Primary Care.* King's Fund, London.

7   Pligt J (1998) Perceived risk and vulnerability as predictors of precautionary behaviour. *Br J Health Psychol.* **3**: 1–14.

8   Department of Health (2000) *An Organisation With a Memory.* Department of Health, London.

9   Reason J (1997) *Managing the Risks of Organisational Accidents.* Ashgate, Aldershot.

Action plan. Module 12: risk management

Today's date: .... Action plan to be completed by: ....

Tackled by	Identify need/assess problem	Plan of action: what will you do?/by when?
Individual – you		
Practice team – you and your colleagues		
Organisation – your practice		

Evaluation: risk management

Complete an evaluation of progress by ....

Level of evaluation: perspective or work done on this component by	The need or problem	Outcome: what have you achieved?	Who was involved in doing it?	Evaluated: • by whom? • when? • what method was used?
Individual – you				
Practice team – you and your colleagues				
Organisation – your practice				

Record of your learning about 'risk management'

Write in topic, date, time spent and type of learning activity

	Activity 1	Activity 2	Activity 3	Activity 4
In-house formal learning				
External courses				
Informal and personal				
Qualifications and/or experience gained				

MODULE 13

Accountability and performance

Clinical governance requires members of the dental team to have robust and effective systems for ensuring the quality of their services. These should meet national clinical standards.

The introduction of quality assurance as part of the Terms of Service for dentists has prompted many dentists to adopt established local accreditation systems in association with the strategic health authority or primary care trust.

They have produced their own local guidelines and standards or modified national standards or guidelines to suit local circumstances. Local quality monitoring has been put in place to detect unacceptable variations in the performance of practices or practitioners. Those responsible for clinical governance should explore the reasons for substandard performance, offer education and practical support, and require action to rectify shortfalls and improve the quality of care for patients.

As health professionals, dentists are accountable to:[1]

- the general public – who are entitled to expect high standards of healthcare
- the profession – to maintain standards of knowledge and skills of the profession as a whole
- the Government – and employers who expect high standards of healthcare from the workforce.

A recent consultation paper seeks to find ways to identify poor performance at an earlier stage in a systematic way.[2] Regular appraisals are seen as being linked into clinical governance and personal development plans, with referral to an assessment and support service for those whose performance is substandard or who have significant health problems.

Accreditation of healthcare

Accreditation of healthcare is a 'means of reviewing the quality of the organisation of health care using external surveyors and published standards'.[3] It is a system of review using external standards. Accreditation systems are mainly found in the USA, Canada and Australia. Standards may be set nationally and checked locally, or set locally and checked by a national body. The results of accreditation may be confidential to the participating organisation, or they may be published to inform the public and purchasers about the performance of local hospitals or health services, especially their levels of success and safety.

Accreditation has been directed at the organisation and management of hospitals rather than the clinical competence of doctors and other health professionals. There are moves to incorporate clinical audit and clinical guidelines into accreditation.[4]

The purpose of accreditation is[5] to:

- improve quality – by stimulating changes in practice
- inform decision making – providing information about performance as guidance
- make healthcare organisations accountable to other statutory agencies or the public
- regulate professional practice and behaviour to protect patients and others.

Accreditation has five key characteristics:[3]

1　review of the performance or capacity to perform (e.g. with respect to a hospital, practice or practitioner)
2　external involvement of a statutory or professional body and/or peers
3　standards concerned with aspects of performance or capacity to be assessed and the values or circumstances that are expected
4　measurement of performance or capacity to perform against those standards
5　report of results – whether performance is at the accepted level, with recommendations for action.

The accreditation programmes available to dentists in primary care include the following:

- ISO accreditation
- Investors in People
- Denplan Excel scheme
- Faculty of General Dental Practitioners' Fellowship by Assessment scheme
- British Dental Association's Good Practice scheme.

Performance assessment framework

The NHS performance assessment framework has six components:[6]

- health improvement
- fair access
- efficiency
- effective delivery of appropriate care
- user experience
- health outcomes.

Working through these in the context of assessing the effectiveness of clinical treatment might mean that you focus on the following.

1   Dental health improvement. You may wish to consider:

  • the impact of your clinical interventions
  • the role of prevention
  • how prevention can be best delivered in your practising circumstances.

2   Fair access to all population groups – matched to needs and circumstances:

  • where and when your practice is open
  • your provision compared with that of other practices.

3   Efficiency:

  • deployment of professional team members
  • value for money.

4   Effective delivery of appropriate care:

  • whether given at the right time by the most appropriate person
  • good knowledge of the availability of other providers in your area.

5   User experience:

  • consistency of messages
  • involvement of parents with those under 16 years of age.

6   Health outcomes – you might focus on any aspect of the outcomes. For example:

  • the oral health score
  • patient perceptions.

Handling underperformance of clinicians

Many health authorities have developed basic screening tools for assessing dentists' performance to detect significant problems of underperformance. Disentangling the performance of a practitioner from that of his or her colleagues or working environment requires a practice visit to scrutinise the individual's performance, practice management and organisational constraints.

The guiding principles for dealing with disciplinary problems among dentists are as follows.

  • Remain non-judgemental; beware of manipulation by others with 'axes to grind'.
  • Be familiar with disciplinary procedures and policies.
  • Document all matters scrupulously, recording objective evidence.
  • Confront the problem and sort it out.
  • Investigate the scope of liaison with representatives of the defence organisation that supports the dentist.

The emphasis in any action plan designed to tackle poor performance should be on education and support rather than a punitive approach to underperformance in the first instance. This approach has been endorsed elsewhere.[7]

One model for GDPs whose performance gives cause for concern might include the following:

- setting up a GDP Support Panel consisting of representatives from the strategic health authority/primary care trust (PCT) and LDC to consider the issues and agree that there are concerns
- conducting a practice visit by up to three members of the Support Panel to assess the situation
- identifying and exploring concerns with the GDP in an attempt to diagnose the causes of the problems
- agreeing a timed action plan – training needs, facilitate learning, feedback, mentorship
- evaluation of progress – the options may be that no further action is required, or there may be ongoing support, a further revised action plan or, in extreme cases, referral to the General Dental Council.

Use of performance indicators in general practice

Performance indicators developed by strategic health authorities/PCTs focus on infra-structure (management, systems, staff time), superstructure (buildings, equipment), educational position (ongoing continuing education) and quality assurance (audit, targets). The focus on structures and procedures is not necessarily related to the quality of clinical care provided, nor does it take into account the patients' perceptions of quality, and variations in provision according to local circumstances and needs.[8]

Indicators commonly used by strategic health authorities when assessing aspects of general practice include the following:

- numbers of complaints
- practice visits
- failure to apply for postgraduate education allowances (PGEA)
- unjustified requests for removal of patients from dental lists
- referral of cases for investigation (e.g. from the Dental Practice Board).

The rigour of external validation may vary from ad hoc surveys and local peer review to involvement in national programmes based on nationally agreed targets for good practice, compliance with which leads to a nationally recognised award. Internal review systems work best when they include monitoring that leads to self-correction where standards slip.

Core values

An exercise in identifying and rating 'core values' for medical practice in the twenty-first century confirmed that patient contact and helping individuals were perceived as key factors.[9] The participants at the conference identified and ranked nine core values in the following order:

1   competence
2   caring
3   commitment
4   integrity
5   compassion
6   responsibility
7   confidentiality
8   spirit of enquiry
9   advocacy.

The same list applies to general dental practice.

Good practice

A recent consultation exercise described the attributes of an 'excellent' GP and one who is 'unacceptable'. Most of these attributes also apply to dental professionals.

The *excellent GP*:[10]

- takes time to listen to patients and allows them to express their concerns
- includes relevant psychological and social factors as well as physical ones
- uses clear and appropriate language for the patient
- is selective but systematic when examining patients
- performs appropriate skilled examinations with consideration for the patient
- has access to necessary equipment and is skilled in its use
- uses investigations where they will help management
- knows about the nature and reliability of investigations, and understands the results
- makes sound management decisions which are based on good practice and evidence
- maintains their knowledge and skills, and is aware of their limits of competence.

The *unacceptable GP* is described as the opposite of most of the above attributes of excellence.

Competence

Responsible clinicians strive to be consciously or unconsciously competent. It is unprofessional to be consciously incompetent or to be unconsciously incompetent where your peers would be expected to have the knowledge and skills to be competent (*see* Figure M13.1).
   A competent clinician will be able to:[11]

- deliver curative and rehabilitative care

	Unconscious	Conscious
Competence	Unconscious competence	Conscious competence
Incompetence	Unconscious incompetence	Unconscious competence

Figure M13.1   Competence of clinicians.

- promote health
- organise preventative health-related activities
- plan, organise and evaluate health education activities
- collaborate with other agents of community development
- participate in research and development
- manage his or her services and resources
- learn with, teach and train other members of the healthcare team
- participate in teamwork
- engage in self-directed learning that is relevant to service needs
- engage in self-evaluation and quality assurance
- be able to demonstrate his or her standards of care and services
- be committed to quality improvement and a clinical governance culture
- involve patients and the public in decision making.

Evidence of competence will include the following:[12]

- well-defined values, functions, responsibilities and direction
- competent management, good leadership, good systems and data, and effective performance monitoring
- a consistent, thorough and systematic approach to practice
- evaluation of the impact of care and procedures
- clear lines of responsibility and accountability
- an overall performance that inspires the confidence and trust of patients and the public.

Quality of care

Clinical governance, professional self-regulation and lifelong learning are the three elements that the Government envisages being cornerstones in achieving high-quality healthcare.[13] The Commission for Health Improvement (CHI) will help to maintain standards of care through its monitoring function. A broad range of performance indicators will be developed through the NHS Performance Framework to identify indicators that are appropriate for effective monitoring of whether care is of high quality.

   The quality of care may be determined by the following:

- timely access to care

- high-quality clinical care (e.g. diagnosis and clinical management)
- high-quality interpersonal care.[2]

The aspects of care that are most highly valued by patients are as follows:[14]

- availability and accessibility of care – appointments, reasonable waiting times, good physical access, ready telephone access
- technical competence – health professional's knowledge and skills, effectiveness of professional's treatment
- communication – time to listen and explain, give information and share in decisions
- interpersonal factors – such as health professional being humane, caring, supportive and trustworthy
- good organisation of care – continuity, co-ordination, near location of services.

Recertification

The introduction of mandatory continuing professional development (lifelong learning) by the GDC is a major development for the dental profession. The key features of this scheme are listed below.

- It applies to all registered dentists.
- It *requires* 250 hours of continuing professional development (CPD) over a five-year period, of which at least 75 hours must be verifiable CPD.
- The *recommendation* is that dentists should normally undertake 50 hours of CPD per year, of which 15 hours should be verifiable.
- It is a statutory scheme to be phased in over three years.
- Dentists can exercise their own judgement as to what they consider to be appropriate CPD.
- All dentists are required to maintain their own CPD records.
- The GDC is to monitor the scheme by random sampling of dentists' records.
- Dentists are to submit annual returns of their CPD hours.
- Failure to comply with lifelong learning may lead to removal from the Dentists' Register.

The benefits of the scheme as described by the GDC are that:

1   it is an opportunity for professional development
2   it allows for greater public protection
3   it formalises existing good practice
4   it is in line with Government policy and other professions.

Making decisions about priorities

When considering the priority to be given to a particular treatment or service, the four dimensions of effectiveness, value, impact and efficiency should be taken into account, as well as the public's preferences and views.[15]

- *Effectiveness* is the extent to which a treatment or other healthcare intervention achieves a desired effect.
- *Value* is a judgement made by an appropriate group as to how valuable that effect is in one patient relative to the value of other treatments.
- *Impact* is the value of an effect weighted for the degree of effectiveness. A treatment or intervention with a high impact will be highly effective, and the effect will be considered very valuable by most people (e.g. extending life by a reasonable amount, substantial reduction of pain, etc.).
- *Efficiency* is the cost of the treatment or intervention for a particular level of impact.

Access to dental services

Other considerations in the prioritising process will relate to equity of access to the healthcare treatment and patient choice. No particular patient group should be discriminated against, even unintentionally. Follow-up monitoring should check that patients receive treatment according to need, and that there are no inequities with regard to age, gender, race, religion, location (e.g. rurality, place of abode), beliefs, learning difficulty, lifestyle, employment status or financial status.

The prioritising group should include a degree of patient choice when considering what alternative treatments to commission, with regard to the expected outcomes of the treatments, the type of interventions and their effects, and the expected benefits for the individual concerned.

These principles have contributed to the drive towards establishing dental access centres, as has the commitment first made by the Prime Minister in September 1999 that by September 2001 anyone would be able to find an NHS dentist simply by calling *NHS Direct*.

In his foreword to *Modernising Dentistry*, Alan Milburn wrote that improving access was a top priority for NHS dentistry. The key features of the dental strategy are as follows:[16]

1 to ensure that everyone should get NHS dentistry if and when they need it – fulfilling the commitment made by the Prime Minister
2 to expand the role of *NHS Direct* so that it can act as a gateway to all NHS dentistry, advising callers on where they can find an NHS dentist and on NHS dental services
3 to develop a modernised and more accessible General Dental Service. Initiatives to achieve this have included:

- up to £4 million in 2000–01 for a Dental Care Development Fund, allowing dental practices to expand and treat more patients

- up to £35 million in 2001–02 to modernise NHS dental practices, providing a better experience for patients and staff alike
- £18 million a year to reward dentists' commitment to the NHS

4 to consider new alternatives to the General Dental Service where it is failing to deliver for patients, including the following:

- projects running around 50 Dental Access Centres, where patients who are not registered with a dentist can receive NHS dental care. The estimate was that access centres would treat up to half a million patients per year
- radical new ways for strategic health authorities to improve the availability of NHS dentistry by entering into contracts with PCTs, independent organisations or individual dentists
- better out-of-hours access for emergency treatment

5 to move dentistry up the NHS agenda, by giving health authorities powerful and flexible new tools for improving access to NHS dentistry, and monitoring their performance

6 to improve the high quality of dental care in the NHS by:

- introducing clinical governance to NHS dentistry, supported by £2 million for individual dental practices and further funding for continuing professional development, clinical audit and peer review
- giving patients easier access to better information about the full range, quality and cost of NHS treatments, and making sure that they are clear about any proposals for private treatment

7 to improve oral health, by providing good advice and information about how to prevent disease, and by reducing inequalities through proactive local schemes aimed at children in particular

8 to invest in improved access to better services.

The Government's commitment to modernising dentistry is reflected in *Options for Change*, a report drawn up by a working group chaired by the then Chief Dental Officer, Dame Margaret Seward.[17] The publication explores a number of areas including professional training, team involvement, workforce implications and new ways of delivering dental services.

Field sites are to be established to pilot different ways of delivering NHS dental services in primary care, and the NHS Modernisation Agency will play a key role in piloting new proposals.

Probity and fraud in the NHS

Fraud is legally defined as involving intentional dishonesty and criminal deception rather than sharp practice or ignorance. The person committing fraud knows that they are breaking the law and gains personally from doing so. Preventing fraud is an activity that straddles corporate and clinical governance. Everyone who works in the NHS has a responsibility to use resources effectively and to guard those resources against fraud, whether they are managers, policy makers, clinicians or non-clinical support staff, through accountability, probity and openness.

Much fraud in the NHS is still thought to be undetected. Prescription fraud alone is estimated to be in excess of £150 million per year in England and Wales.[18] The amount of fraud that was actually detected in the NHS in England and Wales in 1998–99 was £4.7 million, with £3.3 million being in payments for medical services.[19] To put this in context, estimates by the Department of Social Security are of £600 million paid in housing benefits being lost to fraud each year in the UK.[20]

Many of the components of clinical governance will minimise opportunities for fraud in your practice or PCT. As you improve your systems and procedures to guard against errors or omissions in the delivery of patient care, you automatically make it more difficult for people to perpetrate fraud and not be detected. The opportunity to confirm exemption status of patients who are entitled to free treatment under the NHS is one example of recent initiatives in which your team can be involved.

Some examples of the scale of fraud in the NHS[21]

- A patient falsely claimed £2500 a year in travel expenses to an outpatient clinic.
- A pharmacist and GP conspired together to submit bogus prescriptions for reimbursement of over £1 million.
- A dentist falsely claimed £212 000 over two years for patients who did not exist.
- Three opticians falsely claimed £25 000 for supplying tinted glasses.
- A dispensing GP issued bogus prescriptions for patients in residential homes over three years with a value of more than £700 000.
- A GP claimed fees for making 500 night visits in one year against a national average of 50; most of the visits had not been made.

The NHS Counter Fraud Service (CFS) was created in September 1998. Almost 400 counter fraud specialists now work within the NHS. In the three years since its creation, there have been over 90 successful prosecutions (and only one failure), and a 500% increase in monies recovered from the NHS.

The information published in a recent report focuses on dental claims for recalled attendance and domiciliary visits, and is summarised in Figure M13.2.[22]

The Counter Fraud Operational Service (CFOS) has specialist teams working in each of the NHS Regions. There are also local counter fraud specialists sited in each PCT. The counter fraud strategy was outlined in *Countering Fraud in the NHS* and is based on:[23]

- creation of an anti-fraud culture
- maximum deterrence
- successful prevention
- prompt detection
- professional investigation
- effective sanctions
- effective methods of redress.

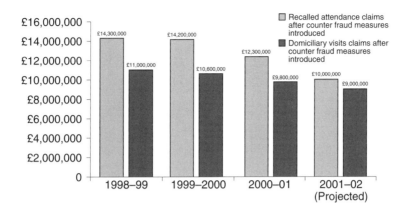

Figure M13.2   Reduced claims from dental contractors after counter fraud measures were introduced.

The Dental Practice Board

The Dental Practice Board (DPB) is a statutory body set up originally under the National Health Service Act 1946, and now under the National Health Service Act 1977 as amended by the Health and Medicines Act 1988.

Its principal functions are as follows:

- approval of payment applications
- calculating and transferring payments
- preventing and detecting fraud and abuse
- providing dental health information.

The DPB also has a duty to ensure that dentists are providing quality treatment, that treatment is provided in accordance with the NHS rules and regulations, and that dentists make accurate claims. Until 1990, the Dental Reference Service, which has been reporting on quality since 1927, was run separately from the probity team, which has been involved in this activity since the 1950s. The merger of activities in 1990 saw an end to the perceived deficiencies of running separate services.

The DPB carries out its duties by:

- performing random and targeted checks on treatment provision or planned treatment through the Dental Reference Service. The DPB aims to examine at least 80 000 randomly selected patients per year, and with its selection process is able to obtain direct clinical evidence of activity of more than 19 out of 20 of the dentists working in the GDS
- sending questionnaires to the patients and comparing the responses with the information provided on the claim forms or by Electronic Data Interchange (EDI). It is checking not only the accuracy of the claim, but also whether patients were given a treatment plan and/or receipt, and how much they were asked to pay
- referral of cases for further investigation if any of the above processes give cause for concern. For example, during the year 1998–99, the DPB referred 197 cases for

consideration of disciplinary action to the health authorities concerned, and a further 15 cases of possible criminal activity were passed to the police.[24]

In addition, the DPB provides each GDS contract holder with an annual prescribing profile that summarises the clinical activity during the preceding 12 months and makes statistical comparisons with peers.

This document, together with a copy of your Dental Reference Officer reports or confirmation from the DPB that the examination of the patient was satisfactory, can contribute to your portfolio of evidence for the purpose of clinical governance.

Some ideas on who should do what about accountability and performance

The GDP

- Be accountable for services in the practice.
- Be accountable for individual patient care.
- Establish methods of proving standards – by a mix of internal and external review.
- Try to live up to the standards of an 'excellent' GDP whenever possible.

The practice manager

- Put systems in place that detect or minimise mistakes or fraudulent practices.
- Check that team members are competent to perform their duties; organise training as necessary.
- Create your own performance indicators in the practice.

The dental nurse

- Co-operate with any performance-monitoring exercise.
- Contribute to assessment of performance by reporting users' experiences.
- Maintain core values.

The receptionist

- Contribute to data collection in any monitoring of systems.
- Adhere to agreed protocols.
- Support the clinical team in reaching and sustaining standards of excellence.
- Keep up to date with current fees and regulations.
- Confirm exemption status by asking to see evidence.

References

1   Grant J, Chambers E and Jackson G (1999) *The Good CPD Guide*. Reed Healthcare, Sutton.

2   Department of Health (1999) *Supporting Doctors, Protecting Patients*. Department of Health, London.

3   Scrivens E (1997) The impact of accreditation systems upon patient care. *J Clin Effect*. **2**.

4   Scrivens E (1998) Policy issues in accreditation. *Int J Qual Health Care*. **10**: 1–5.

5   Walshe K, Walsh N, Schofield T and Blakeway-Phillips C (eds) (2000) *Accreditation in Primary Care: towards clinical governance*. Radcliffe Medical Press, Oxford.

6   NHS Executive (1999) *The NHS Performance Assessment Framework*. Department of Health, London.

7   GPs Performance Project Steering Group (1997) *Screening and Educational Assessment*. South Thames Deanery, London.

8   Birch K, Scrivens E and Field S (1998) *Quality in Primary Care*. University of Keele, Keele.

9   British Medical Association (1995) *Core Values for the Medical Profession in the 21st century*. British Medical Association, London.

10 Royal College of General Practitioners/General Practitioners Committee (2002) *Good Medical Practice for General Practitioners*. RCGP, GPC, London.

11 Southgate L (1994) Freedom and discipline: clinical practice and the assessment of clinical competence. *Br J Gen Pract*. **44**: 87–92.

12 Irvine D (1997) The performance of doctors. 1. Professionalism and self-regulation in a changing world. *BMJ*. **314**: 1540–2.

13 NHS Executive (1999) *Quality and Performance in the NHS: clinical indicators*. NHS Executive, Leeds.

14 Roland M (1999) Quality and efficiency: enemies or partners? *Br J Gen Pract*. **49**: 140–3.

15 Rajaratnum G (1999) *Prioritising Health and Health Care in North Staffordshire: a proposal to establish a North Staffordshire Priorities Forum*. North Staffordshire Health Authority, Stoke-on-Trent.

16 Department of Health (2000) *Modernising NHS Dentistry. Implementing the NHS Plan*. The Stationery Office, London.

17 Department of Health (2002) *Options for Change*. The Stationery Office, London.

18 NHS Executive (1997) *Prescription Fraud. An efficiency scrutiny*. NHS Executive, London.

19 Audit Commission (1999) *Protecting the Public Purse: ensuring probity in the NHS*. Audit Commission, London.

20 Accounts Commission for Scotland (1998) *Annual Report*. Accounts Commission for Scotland, Edinburgh.

21 NHS Executive (1998) *Countering Fraud in the NHS*. NHS Executive, Leeds.

22 Department of Health (2002) *Countering Fraud in the NHS: protecting resources for patients, 1998–2001 performance statistics*. The Stationery Office, London.

23 Department of Health (1998) *Countering Fraud in the NHS*. The Stationery Office, London.

24 Dental Practice Board (1998) *Annual Review 1998–99*. Dental Practice Board, Eastbourne.

Action plan. Module 13: accountability and performance

Today's date: ....   Action plan to be completed by: ....

Tackled by	Identify need/assess problem	Plan of action: what will you do?/by when?
Individual – you		
Practice team – you and your colleagues		
Organisation – your practice		

Evaluation: accountability and performance

Complete an evaluation of progress by ....

Level of evaluation: perspective or work done on this component by	The need or problem	Outcome: what have you achieved?	Who was involved in doing it?	Evaluated: • by whom? • when? • what method was used?
Individual – you				
Practice team – you and your colleagues				
Organisation – your practice				

Record of your learning about 'accountability and performance'

Write in topic, date, time spent and type of learning activity

	Activity 1	Activity 2	Activity 3	Activity 4
In-house formal learning				
External courses				
Informal and personal				
Qualifications and/or experience gained				

MODULE 14

Core requirements

Clinical governance will be a challenge for all members of the dental team. It requires a shift in culture, in particular:

- education and training focused on organisational needs and on the needs of the individual
- adequate resources to provide time both for the work and for the training
- the identification and development of leadership
- the development of a 'no-blame' culture within the practice.

If we revert to the big picture for a moment, the NHS Performance Assessment Framework[1] requires health authorities, primary care groups and NHS trusts working with social services departments to use the Framework to assess local performance, support the development of the local Health Improvement Programmes and account to ministers and the public for performance. This will be done by means of the following:

- assessing overall performance using the six areas of the framework (*see* Module 13 on Accountability and performance)
- comparing service development over time, benchmarking the services with other similar organisations, assessing the reasons for variation and the scope for local improvements, using these comparisons for developing and agreeing local action plans
- incorporating, in future performance and accountability agreements and monitoring arrangements, an assessment of actual and planned progress in the six areas.

The document[1] also recognises that the local delivery of high-quality healthcare is underpinned by modernised professional self-regulation and extended lifelong learning.

We need the right staff and the right resources in the right place at the right time.

In this Module we shall consider the following topics:

- training and competence
- right skill mix
- safe and comfortable environment
- cost-effectiveness.

Training and competence

1   Staff need to be:

- appropriately qualified to do the job when appointed (*see* Module 2 on Managing resources and services) *or*
- correctly trained to an assessed competence before being allowed to work without supervision.

2   Every staff member should have a personal and professional development plan supported by the practice principal or partners.

3   Identify staff education and training needs (not wants) according to:

- the requirements of the practice
- identified individual deficiencies in knowledge, skills or attitudes.

4   Education and training should be provided in-house or elsewhere, and the time to do this should be supported.

Review performance continuously by audit to establish competence and identify attitude problems or gaps in knowledge or skills.

See also Module 8 on Coherent teamwork.

Risk management is not a blame-and-shame culture. People should feel comfortable about revealing their own or other people's mistakes (*see* Module 12 on Risk management).

We must collect *meaningful* quality measures (*see also* Module 4 on Reliable and accurate data).

Crude referral rates are unhelpful. A high rate can conceal gaps in knowledge, skills or resources. a low rate may indicate poor knowledge of secondary facilities or insufficient knowledge of diagnosis. High rates may be due to special interest or demographic peculiarities. Low rates may be due to extensive provision for the condition in primary care.

The same applies to some extent to the information contained in the annual prescribing profiles sent out to GDS dentists each year by the Dental Practice Board. The analyses may be an indicator of trends or prescribing preferences, but comparisons can be futile if the specific practising circumstances of individuals are not taken into account.

Right skill mix

People perform inappropriate tasks for the following reasons.

- It has always been done that way.
- There is no one else to do it.
- No one has thought about the best way to do it.
- They enjoy doing that job.

Delegation or enhancement

Consider delegation to others who are less expensively paid or less extensively trained. For example, it makes no sense for a dentist to be spending time investigating stock control, when the task can be delegated to a team member with a little training. As well as being less expensive, the quality of the service may be better, as someone who is concentrating on one task tends to be more skilful.

The skill mix present in any team is very wide.

Start by finding out what the patients need, then what the service needs, and then plan for the people you need to meet those needs – what one paper[2] calls 'reprofiling and aligning skills with organisational needs' for workforce planning.

For other information on skill mix, *see* Module 8 on Coherent teamwork.

Safe and comfortable environment

A Health Service Circular[3] reminds us all of good practice with regard to the health, safety and welfare of NHS staff. Managers are responsible for ensuring that they:

*   comply with health and safety legislation – there is a lack of knowledge and understanding, and compliance can be seriously lacking[4]
*   assess risk and, where practicable, eliminate it
*   integrate health and safety with mainstream management (i.e. do not *just* delegate it to a member of staff)
*   ensure that there is a partnership between the practice and outside agencies and individuals
*   set audit standards for the organisation and conduct an audit regularly.

Think about risk management in as wide a context as possible. It is not just about avoiding complaints, but also about making the working conditions safe and comfortable. Look at Module 2 on Managing resources and services. All new team members need an induction pack that includes health and safety recommendations and advice on risk avoidance. This includes the promotion of best practice. Module 5 on Evidence-based practice and policy looks at many aspects of good-quality care.

Guidelines on best practice for the prevention of cross-infection between patients are available from a variety of organisations. For example, the British Dental Association has produced an advice sheet on the subject jointly with the Department of Health. A discussion with the team on how best to implement the guidelines should enable the latter to be put into practice. If the practical difficulties are too great, then the team needs to be able to report those difficulties to someone who can remedy the situation.

Although comparable studies are not available for dentistry, it is interesting to note that an article published in 1995[5] found that 85% of general practices in the Liverpool area (74.5% response rate) did not have a written infection control policy. Autoclaves were used in 80% of practices, but most did not have any written procedures for their use. Few practices had any information about procedures for infected patients or staff. One-third had no policy on needlestick injuries, and sharps incidents were recorded in less than half of the surgeries. This prompted training and the development of guidelines focused on the practice nurses. There is anecdotal evidence that this is not as widespread a problem in general dental practice, because many practices have been the subject of in-depth practice visits by the health authority's nominated person(s).

Staff training

This should:

- raise awareness of clinical risk management
- include specific training in adverse incident reporting and indicate to whom staff should report their concerns
- avoid a blame culture
- include training for those collecting and evaluating data
- show staff how to promote best practice themselves.

Review and control of hazards

This may include:

- a meeting with the staff concerned to discover the problems
- consideration of staffing levels or skill mix
- training for the work or for avoidance of risk
- developing and implementing protocols and guidelines
- checking building and equipment for suitability and safety
- reporting unsafe practices, equipment or buildings
- seeking expert advice.

An agency nurse found that the surgery sharps container was frequently left on a low table and was often filled above the maximum level. She left notes for the regular staff, but they were ignored. At a meeting concerning something else, she raised her concerns. An investigation found that the responsibility for sharps boxes had been delegated to a member of staff who was absent on long-term sick leave. Everyone else thought it was someone else's job! Information about the procedure for sharps disposal was disseminated. Each nurse who set up the surgery was given responsibility for renewing and storage of the sharps containers.

Safety is not just about safely constructed and maintained buildings and a clear fire exit. The personal safety of staff is extremely important. The design and use of a building can minimise dangerous situations.

Enable staff to receive training in recognising the early signs of threat, and in how to avoid or defuse confrontations.

Comfort and good health at work include the management and control of excess stress. Common causes of mental distress are lack of control over workload or working standards, and lack of appreciation of work well done.

Poor mental health and high stress levels have been reported in staff working in general practice. Around 65% of general practitioners felt that stress had caused mistakes in their practices. Support from colleagues, time for reflection and discussion as well as avoidance of work overload were all shown to be important factors in preventing burnout.

Cost-effectiveness

Cost-effectiveness is not synonymous with 'cheapness'. A cost-effective intervention is one which gives a better or equivalent benefit from the intervention in question for lower or equivalent cost, or where the relative improvement in outcome is higher than the relative difference in cost. In other words, being cost-effective means having the best outcomes for the least input. Using the term 'cost-effective' implies that you have considered potential alternatives.

An intervention must first be considered to be *clinically* effective to warrant investigation into its potential to be *cost*-effective. Evidence-based practice must incorporate clinical judgement. You have to interpret the evidence when it comes to applying it to individual patients, whether it be evidence about clinical effectiveness or about cost-effectiveness.

If you want to ask a question about cost-effectiveness, you should be sure to have confirmed clinical effectiveness first, and have gone on to ask a question about cost-effectiveness as the second stage in seeking the evidence. A new or alternative treatment or intervention should be compared directly with the next best treatment or intervention.

An economic evaluation is a comparative analysis of two or more alternatives in terms of their costs and consequences. There are four different types:

1   cost-effectiveness
2   cost minimisation
3   cost utility
4   cost–benefit analyses.

Cost-effectiveness analysis is used to compare the effectiveness of two interventions with the same treatment objectives. Cost minimisation compares the costs of alternative treatments which have identical health outcomes. Cost utility analysis enables the effects of alternative interventions to be measured against a combination of life expectancy and quality of life. A cost–benefit analysis compares the incremental cost and benefits of a programme.

Efficiency is sometimes confused with effectiveness. Being efficient means obtaining the most quality from the least expenditure, or the required level of quality for the least expenditure. To measure efficiency you need to make a judgement about the level of quality of the 'purchase' and be able to relate it to 'price'. 'Price' alone does not measure efficiency. Quality is the indicator used in combination with price to assess whether something is more efficient.

Thus, cost-effectiveness is a measure of efficiency and suggests that costs have been related to effectiveness.

If you have a finite budget to spend, it is inescapable that expenditure in one area of your practice will mean less in another. Many team members are reluctant to become involved in any financial decision making. They entered the practice with altruistic motives that did not include having to make difficult decisions about value for money.

Giving people control over their own small budgets and making them aware of the relative costs of equipment and materials can be useful. It gives people the information that they need in order to take control of how they use supplies, treatments or technologies.

Considerable uncertainty exists with regard to attempting to work out how to compare interventions in terms of the extra cost per unit of health outcome obtained, because:

1   health economists are still debating the methodological framework underlying the decisions
2   the data are uncertain because:

  •   assumptions are made in different ways
  •   data are missing
  •   the data are interpreted in different ways

3   the presentation and interpretation of the results are often subjective or biased.

The types of costs involved in studies of cost-effectiveness include those shown in the table opposite.

Even if they are valid in a descriptive sense, these measures may not be suitable for economic evaluation.

Health service costs	Non-health service costs	Other costs
Costs of the study	Costs incurred in other public sector budgets, such as social services	Transfer costs where money flows from one group in society to another (e.g. from taxes to social security payments)
Direct costs of the intervention	Informal care costs	
Costs of treating other illnesses arising from the intervention	Patients' travel costs	
Costs of treating other unrelated illnesses discovered during the intervention study	Other out-of-pocket expenses incurred by patients	
Future costs incurred because of any lengthening of life resulting from the intervention	Patients' time costs taken up by the intervention	
	Productivity and work time costs taken up by the intervention	
	Future costs incurred because of any lengthening of life resulting from the intervention	

Some ideas on who should do what to strengthen core requirements

Many of the core requirements will be covered by activities in other modules.

The GDP

*   Be pro-active about changing skill mix.
*   Be responsible for monitoring cost-effective information.
*   Monitor outcomes of care.

The practice manager

*   Establish clear lines of accountability.
*   Take overall responsibility for employing well-trained and competent staff.
*   Support staff.
*   Be responsible for the safety and comfort of staff.

The dental nurse

- Pursue reflective practice around skill mix.
- Give feedback to others on patient experience.

The receptionist

- Report safety hazards.
- Relay feedback from patients.
- Ensure fair access to health professionals and services.
- Maintain competence and professional standards.

References

1   Department of Health (1999) *The NHS Performance Assessment Framework.* Department of Health, London.

2   Gill P (1996) The importance of workforce planning in the NHS in the 1990s. *Health Man Manage.* **22**: 21–5.

3   Department of Health (1998) *Management of Health Safety and Welfare Issues for NHS Staff.* Department of Health, London.

4   Sen D and Osborne K (1997) General practices and health and safety at work. *Br J Gen Pract.* **47**: 103–4.

5   White RR and Smith JM (1995) Infection control in general practice: results of a questionnaire survey. *J Pub Health.* **17**: 146–9.

Action plan. Module 14: core requirements

Today's date: .... Action plan to be completed by: ....

Tackled by	Identify need/assess problem	Plan of action: what will you do?/by when?
Individual – you		
Practice team – you and your colleagues		
Organisation – your practice		

Evaluation: core requirements

Complete an evaluation of progress by ....

Level of evaluation: perspective or work done on this component by	The need or problem	Outcome: what have you achieved?	Who was involved in doing it?	Evaluated: • by whom? • when? • what method was used?
Individual – you				
Practice team – you and your colleagues				
Organisation – your practice				

Record of your learning about 'core requirements'

Write in topic, date, time spent and type of learning activity

	Activity 1	Activity 2	Activity 3	Activity 4
In-house formal learning				
External courses				
Informal and personal				
Qualifications and/or experience gained				

PART THREE

Quality improvement

The challenges of
quality improvement

We know that clinical governance is a new name for joining together many things that we already do to a greater or lesser degree. It is a framework for the improvement of patient care through achieving high standards, reflective practice and risk management, as well as personal and professional development. The corollary is that the enhancement of quality of care is based on each and every module in this book.

The challenges of definition

'Quality' is a key word in any statement about clinical governance, but there are many definitions of the word. If you look in a dictionary you will find that the word means:

- a characteristic or attribute of something; a property; a feature
- the natural or essential character of something
- the degree or grade of excellence
- excellence or superiority.

Roy Lilley[1] defines it as 'knowing what outcome you want and being sure you get it, every time, for as long as you want it'.

The purpose of clinical governance is to shift the standard of care towards better quality. In Figure 1 overleaf, each bell-shaped curve represents the pattern of clinical performance at any one time. The pattern of performance by each practice or the clinical output of each clinician will follow the normal distribution curve, with most people performing to an adequate standard most of the time. There will be episodes of suboptimal performance along the way (denoted by the double-headed arrow) within the quality zone. The purpose of clinical governance is to shift the mean standard of care (denoted by the dotted line) through the range of activities described in this book, and each complete cycle of activity should facilitate this. By the time the third cycle is complete, the mean standard of care will have improved. Not only does this model apply to individual practice, but it is equally applicable to general practice as a whole, where the shift can be brought about by better dissemination of information relating to, say, evidence-based dentistry.

There are four broad perspectives on quality, which fall into the following categories:

1   professional
2   lay

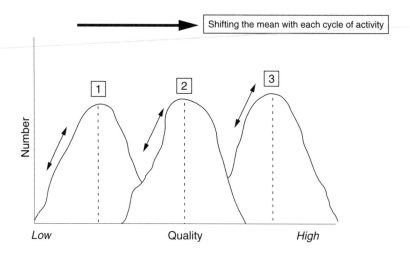

Figure 1   Cycles of performance.

3   managerial
4   political.

Professional perspective

The professional perspective on quality has been driven by competency-based assessments and reviewing performance in relation to current standards, guidelines and protocols.

In the current climate of accountability, the conduct and performance of professionals are under increasing scrutiny. Media coverage focused on the Bristol heart surgery case, the Shipman Inquiry and the Melvyn Megitt case in dentistry has helped to maintain the media's interest in the professions, and has brought the quality debate into the public arena.

Lay perspective

The needs and expectations of the patient will alter the precise definition of quality. The service provided must fit the needs of the user within the constraints of cost and present levels of knowledge and technology.[1] The priority then must be to understand the needs of the users and then (and only then) to provide for these.

We know from experience that patients do not always want to know or even care how we prepare a crown, or the technical details of its laboratory construction, but we also know that they are aware of the quality of the 'process' which leads to delivering the benefit of that treatment.

Managerial and political perspectives

The managerial and political perspective has been related to cost and activity. The Department of Health has put forward its view on quality, which states that:

> Every part of the NHS and everyone who works in it should take responsibility for working to improve quality. This must be quality in its broadest sense, doing the right things at the right time for the right people, and doing them right – first time. And it must be the quality of the patient's experience as well as the clinical result – quality measured in terms of prompt access, good relationships and efficient administration.[2]

From a management perspective, five universal dimensions of this quality can be identified:[3]

1   dependability – did the provider do what was promised?
2   responsiveness – was the service provided in a timely manner?
3   authority – did the provider elicit a feeling of confidence in the customer during the service delivery process?
4   empathy – was the service provider able to take the customer's point of view?
5   tangible evidence – was evidence left that the service was indeed performed?

It is a fact that all of those involved in the delivery of healthcare tend to emphasise the value of the particular parts of the care process that are central to their particular role.

If quality is defined in partial terms, separating out any of these aspects from another will give priority to one particular view – and it may not be the one that improves the quality of care for the patient.

Components of quality care

The components of quality care can be conveniently broken down into the areas of technical expertise of service delivery and those areas which relate to the quality of the practice–patient interface and the professional–patient encounter. These can be subdivided into aspects of structure, process and outcome in a development of the Donabedian model.

See Module 9 on Audit and evaluation.

	Structure (resources)	Process (activities)	Outcome (results)
Effectiveness	Do staff qualifications/ training conform with current requirements?	Are best practice guidelines and protocols adhered to?	
Acceptability	To what extent are the facilities judged satisfactory by users?		Is the outcome of treatment acceptable to patients?
Efficiency			How do the fixed and variable costs compare with other practices?
Access (part of the big picture)		What proportion of the total population that is in need of treatment receives it and after how long?	
Equity		Is there bias in access between social groups?	
Relevance	Do staff deployments match the patterns of expressed consumer need?		Is there a health gain resulting from treatment that could be generated by alternatives (prevention)?

Challenges of measurement

Those facets of the health service that are easiest to quantify are not always the most important ones.[4]

If a patient uses the subjective measure as being indicative of quality provision, they are not necessarily reading it right. Speaking at the annual Dental Practice Board Conference in April 2001, Chris Morris (a dentally qualified partner at Hempsons Solicitors) noted that 'the patient's judgement of the quality of the treatment will be a subjective one, and a second professional opinion of that treatment may or may not be an objective one'. The challenge of meaningful measurement remains.

There is no reason why qualitative measures[5] should not be used alongside quantitative ones. In the past, failures to appreciate the importance of using appropriate measurements have acted as barriers to improvements. Attempts at measurement have been simplistic and often crude because the processes frequently fail to recognise all of the relevant factors.

There is a view that quality cannot be assessed. 'It is important to establish that it is theoretically possible to evaluate quality, otherwise all effort will be in vain. The definition of quality states that it is the property of judgement on care ... The confusion over the nature of quality arises from the difficulty of explaining the reasons for the presence or absence of quality.'[6]

It was suggested (*see* Module 9 on Audit and evaluation) that the approach to quality is likely to be based on a hierarchical approach ranging from a number of essential to desirable indicators. If this approach is extrapolated, one suitable hierarchical model could look like that shown in Figure 2.

Practice involvement in quality	Examples of what this might mean
Practice has been externally validated	The practice has completed the national programme but has also achieved additional accreditation through the Fellowship by Assessment from the FGDP or Investors in People or ISO 9000
Completion of national programme	The practice has completed a nationally recognised scheme
Active involvement in national programme	The practice is involved in a nationally recognised scheme such as the BDA's Good Practice Scheme, or is involved in vocational training
Active involvement in a quality assurance programme	The practice is aware of current issues and adopts a proactive stance on the quality assurance agenda
Statutory and desirable measures in place	The practice complies with legislation but also has in place some desirable systems of quality assurance over and above the essential requirements
Statutory quality measures all in place	The practice has been visited by the health authority and is able to demonstrate compliance with essential legislation
Some quality measures in place	The practice has some elements of essential requirements in place, but there are also some areas which require attention
Lacking strategic direction	The practice operates on an informal basis with little regard for current trends and low awareness of current issues

Figure 2 A suggested hierarchical model of quality initiatives in general dental practice, based on a model proposed by Birch *et al.*[7]

Who decides?

The requirements of quality of treatment expected from a dentist under the NHS are set out in the Terms of Service. Those who decide whether that standard has been met include Dental Reference Officers, the Dental Practice Board Probity Unit, the Dental Disciplinary Committee, the Health Services Appeal Authority and the NHS tribunals. In summary, a mixture of dentists, lawyers and lay people decide whether the NHS quality standards have been met.[8]

The quality standard in criminal courts may be decided by the police/crown prosecution service, a jury, a Court of Appeal or the House of Lords. The standard of proof is 'beyond reasonable doubt'. In contrast, the standard of proof in civil courts is one of 'balance of probability', and it will be determined by judges assisted by dental experts where necessary.

The quality standard expected by the General Dental Council is decided by the Preliminary Proceedings Committee and the Professional Conduct Committee.

Ultimately, practitioners must take 100% responsibility for the quality of care that they provide and 'in 100% of situations it is the patient who is the most important person to judge that quality'.[8]

As the management gurus have been saying for a long time, 'any decision about quality which fails to take into account the customer is immediately suspect'.

The patient is a consumer of dental services. Because patient perceptions of quality and value are relative, effective service delivery requires the adaptation of services to individual needs.[9] Aspects of service quality have been discussed in Module 9 on Audit and evaluation.

Challenges of where and how to deliver care

Looking at the big picture again, the provision of healthcare in the broadest sense can be analysed at three distinct levels.

1   At the community level, involving care for the whole population. Taxation or insurance schemes fund equitable levels of care for all. The system is run through official bureaucracy and is politically based.
2   At the institutional or managerial level, by a particular hospital or practice serving part of a population. The user or their agent chooses the particular unit or service provided.
3   At the practice or individual professional level, where it is usually focused on the interests of particular patients. It is driven by peer-group pressure, ethics and moral values.

Much of health promotion activity has to be done at the first, political level (see Module 11 on Health promotion), and resources can be directed to particular areas for clinical care. Efficiency of care and service improvements have typically occurred at Level 2, and clinical effectiveness and personal care at Level 3.

Delivery of quality care in general dental practice has been marked by conflicts between these levels. We need to find effective ways of working co-operatively to produce quality improvements.

The challenge of how to deal with poor quality

There is a prevailing management perspective that exploiting fear of punishment is the only way to get things done. All of the evidence suggests that this produces defensiveness and concealment of difficulties and errors. The logic of management requires attitudes that support rather than punish (*see* Module 2 on Managing resources and services), and recognition that most people wish to work well and assist those around them.

The challenge of who the health service is for

Let us not lose sight of the patients in the management of healthcare. In general dental practices, business pressures can force decision making in which the patient becomes part of the 'market', and commercial pressures may dictate which market segment any particular practice aims to cater for. The challenge for the health service is to retain and support sufficient resources to make provision for the marketplace in its entirety.

Challenges of resources

It must be said that very little has been offered to support clinical governance in general dental practice. That is abundantly clear. We know that it is an integral part of our daily work, but it does not come without investment in time and costs.

It is fallacious to suggest that clinical governance will result in overall savings on cost, but it may be true that it will produce a more profitable business environment, given its close links with the principles of good management. However, not everyone agrees with this perspective. Whatever the outcome of that particular debate, it must be recognised that quality does not come free of charge.

A challenge for the future

We have all heard or seen examples of excellence in primary dental care. The challenge is to move from establishing minimum reasonable standards for care to identifying customary standards and then to recommended best practice.

This is what most GDPs want to do each time we go into our practices.

So what is new if we are already talking the talk and walking the walk?

The answer lies in the footprints of clinical governance.

References

1   Lilley R (2000) *Making Sense of Clinical Governance* (revised edition). Radcliffe Medical Press, Oxford.

2   Department of Health (1997) *The New NHS: modern, dependable*. The Stationery Office, London.

3   Parasuraman A, Zeithaml V and Berry L (1988) SERVQUAL: a multiple-item scale for measuring consumer perceptions of service quality. *J Retail*. **Spring**: 12–40.

4   Donnan S (1998) The health of adult Europe: combating inequalities involves measuring what counts. *BMJ*. **316**: 1620–1.

5   Cleary PD (1997) Subjective and objective measures of health: which is better when? *J Health Serv Res Policy*. **2**: 3–4.

6   Baker R (1992) *Practice Assessment and Quality of Care*. Royal College of General Practitioners, London.

7   Birch K, Field S and Scrivens E (2000) *Quality in General Practice*. Radcliffe Medical Press, Oxford.

8   Dental Practice Board (2000) *DPB Dental Conference Report*. Dental Practice Board, Eastbourne.

9   Heskett JL, Sasser WE and Schlesinger LA (1997) *The Service Profit Chain*. Simon & Schuster, New York.

Appendix: resources

Useful websites

Bandolier: http://www.jr2.ox.ac.uk/bandolier/index.html

Centre for Evidence-Based Medicine (CEBM): http://cebm.jr2.ox.ac.uk/

Clinical Evidence from the British Medical Journal Publishing Group: http://www.evidence.org

Cochrane Library, Update Software Ltd, Summertown Pavilion, Middle Way, Summertown, Oxford OX2 7LG: http://www.cochrane.co.uk

Database of Abstracts of Reviews of Effectiveness (DARE) contains high-quality research reviews of the effectiveness of healthcare interventions: http://nhscrd.york.ac.uk/welcome.html

E-learning initiatives for the dental team: www.smile-on.com

Guidelines database containing a summary, a detailed critical appraisal of the quality and robustness, and a link to the detailed document: http://www.his.ox.ac.uk/guidelines/

Medline: http://www.ncbi.nlm.nih.gov/PubMed

OMNI (use the search facility for dental links and references): http://www.omni.ac.uk

Practice management information: www.first-practice.com

PubMed National Library of Medicine search service to access Medline with links to allied journals: http://www4.ncbi.nlm.gov/PubMed

ScHaRR Introduction to Free Databases: http://www.shef.ac.uk/~scharr/ir/trawling.html

smile-on.com: an online introductory clinical governance course.

Steve's Attempt To Teach Statistics (STATS) contains useful information on statistics and their interpretation: http://www.cmh.edu/stats

WISDOM (part of the Institute of General Practice and Primary Care, University of Sheffield): http://www.wisdom.org.uk

Useful publications on evidence-based practice and clinical effectiveness

Bandolier This is published by the NHS Executive, Anglia and Oxford, as a monthly newsletter that describes the literature on the effectiveness of healthcare interventions in a pithy style. Moore A and McQuay H (eds) *Bandolier*, Pain Relief Unit, The Churchill, Oxford OX3 7LJ. http://www.jr2.ox.ac.uk/Bandolier

Clinical Effectiveness Resource Pack This resource pack is updated regularly and is produced by the NHS Executive. It includes lists of contact details for many organisations, and lists of publications and other sources of information on clinical effectiveness. There is also information about associated publications, including the Effective Health Care Bulletins, Effectiveness Matters, Epidemiologically Based Needs Assessments, Systematic Reviews of Research Evidence, Clinical Guidelines, Health Technology Assessments and other relevant publications.

Clinical Evidence A twice-yearly compendium of the best available evidence for effective healthcare. BMJ Publishing Group. Launched in 1999.

Effective Healthcare Bulletins These bulletins are produced by the NHS Centre for Reviews and Dissemination at the University of York. They are 'based on systematic review and synthesis of research on the clinical effectiveness, cost-effectiveness and acceptability of health service interventions'. NHS Centre for Reviews and Dissemination, University of York, York YO1 5DD. Subscriptions and copies are available from Royal Society of Medicine Press, PO Box 9002, London W1A 0ZA.

He@lth Information on the Internet This is a bimonthly newsletter for all healthcare professionals, published by the Royal Society of Medicine in association with the Wellcome Trust. He@lth Information on the Internet, Royal Society of Medicine, 1 Wimpole Street, London W1M 8AE. Tel: 020 7290 2927.

Health Updates from the Health Development Agency. Topics in the series include Coronary Heart Disease, Smoking, Alcohol, Physical Activity, Workplace Health, Child Health and Immunisation. These are well-researched reference books on topical health issues. Health Updates, Health Development Agency, Trevelyan House, 30 Great Peter Street, London SW1P 2HW.

Relevant books

Armstrong R and Grace J (1994) *Research Methods and Audit in General Practice*. Oxford University Press, Oxford.

British Dental Association (1999) *BDA Clinical Governance Kit*. British Dental Association, London.

Carter Y and Thomas C (eds) (1997) *Research Methods in Primary Care.* Radcliffe Medical Press, Oxford.

Chambers R and Boath E (2001) *Clinical Effectiveness and Clinical Governance Made Easy* (2e). Radcliffe Medical Press, Oxford.

Chambers R (2000) *Involving Patients and the Public: how to do it better.* Radcliffe Medical Press, Oxford.

Chambers R and Wall D (2000) *Teaching Made Easy: a manual for health professionals.* Radcliffe Medical Press, Oxford.

Crombie I (1996) *The Pocket Guide to Critical Appraisal.* BMJ Publishing Group, London.

Faculty of General Dental Practitioners (1992) *SAMS Manual: self-assessment manual and standards.* Faculty of General Dental Practitioners, London.

Gillies A (2002) *Providing Information for Health: a workbook for primary care.* Radcliffe Medical Press, Oxford.

Gray JAM (1997) *Evidence-Based Healthcare.* Churchill Livingstone, Edinburgh.

Greenhalgh T (1997) *How to Read a Paper: the basics of evidence-based medicine.* BMJ Publishing Group, London.

Jones R and Kinmonth AL (eds) (1999) *Critical Reading for Primary Care.* Oxford University Press, London.

King's Fund (1998) *Turning Evidence into Everyday Practice.* King's Fund, London.

Lilley R (2000) *Making Sense of Clinical Governance* (revised edition). Radcliffe Medical Press, Oxford.

Lilley R with Lambden P (2000) *Making Sense of Risk Management* (revised edition). Radcliffe Medical Press, Oxford.

Lugon M and Secker-Walker J (1999) *Clinical Governance: making it happen.* Royal Society of Medicine Press, London.

Newsome P (2001) *The Patient-Centred Practice. A practical guide to customer care.* BDJ Books, London.

NHS Executive (1996) *Patient Partnership: building a collaborative strategy.* NHS Executive, Leeds.

Pike S and Forster D (1995) *Health Promotion for All.* Churchill Livingstone, Edinburgh. (This book contains a framework for developing a personal health promotion portfolio.)

Rattan R (1996) *Making Sense of Dental Practice Management.* Radcliffe Medical Press, Oxford.

Rattan R (2002) *Vocational Training in General Dental Practice: a handbook for trainers.* Radcliffe Medical Press, Oxford.

Tyrrell S (2002) *Using the Internet in Healthcare* (2e). Radcliffe Medical Press, Oxford.

van Zwanenberg T and Harrison J (eds) (2000) *Clinical Governance in Primary Care.* Radcliffe Medical Press, Oxford.

Wakley G, Chambers R and Field S (2000) *Continuing Professional Development in Primary Care.* Radcliffe Medical Press, Oxford.

Wilson T (ed.) (1999) *The PCG Development Guide.* Radcliffe Medical Press, Oxford.

Index